The
Metabolic
Makeover

It's all about energy.

STEPHEN CHERNISKE
& NATALIE KATHER, M.D.

The purpose of this book is to educate,
not to diagnose or prescribe.

ISBN-13: 978-1493707485
ISBN-10: 1493707485

Design/illustration by April Sunset
www.fuseologycreative.com

Manufactured in the United States.

First Edition: January 2014

Table of Contents

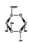

Table of Contents (cont'd)

Dedication

To Linus Pauling, Rosalind Franklin, James Watson and Francis Crick. Together, these brilliant scientists discovered the structure of DNA, which made this book, and your transformation possible.

Acknowledgements

If we listed all the scientists we are indebted to, the acknowledgements would take up half the book. Let us just say that every scientific advance is a group effort. The fact that this book contains more than 200 references is an indication of the degree to which we build on the insights and discoveries of others. Natalie and I are simply doing our part.

I am certainly indebted to Bill Lee for putting his money where my mouth is. Mr. Lee's sponsorship of critical research for more than two decades is testimony to his world vision and remarkable generosity.

Like to thank Stephen Hicks at Hobby Street Studios for his hard work on mastering an audio masterpiece with our audiobook.

Then there is the hard work of bringing a manuscript and brand to life, expertly handled by April Sunset and Michael Paul at FuseologyCreative.com, along with Jim Kreinbrink and Barbara Bischoff.

About the Authors

Stephen Cherniske, M.S. is a biochemist and former university instructor in Clinical Nutrition. He served on the faculty of the American College of Sports Medicine, advised members of the US Olympic team, and directed the nation's first federally licensed clinical laboratory specializing in nutrition and immunology. A best-selling author with more than a million copies in print, Stephen has a remarkable gift for communicating breakthrough science that inspires, entertains and motivates.

Natalie Kather, M.D. received her medical degree from The University of Utah School of Medicine. She is board-certified in Family Medicine, as well as Anti-aging, with specialties in women's health, hormone balancing and human performance. Natalie is recognized as a pioneer in the emerging science of metabolic medicine, and frequently serves as Principal Investigator for clinical trials in that arena. Her clinic, Advanced Family Wellness, is located in Olympia Washington, where she lives with her husband, Stephen Cherniske.

Introduction

I boarded a flight to Seattle five years ago and, as usual, took out my laptop to work. A diagram of a glycogen molecule appeared on my screen, which intrigued the woman next to me. I explained that glycogen is one of the ways that animals, including humans, store energy. "Why are you working with glycogen?" she asked. Not wanting to get drawn into a lengthy discussion, I simply replied, "It's part of something I call *The Metabolic Makeover.*"

"I want that," she said.

"I haven't even told you what it is," I replied. Then she surprised me. "I don't care," she said, "I want a metabolic makeover." It was then that I realized this book had to be written.

Everyone wants a metabolic makeover, because everyone is aware that it has something to do with quality of life, weight management, and energy. Everyone I talked to after that experience agreed – (before even having the details) that if they could safely and effectively improve their metabolism, that would be a very good thing.

Natalie and I developed *The Metabolic Makeover* program in 2011. Since then, it has vastly improved the quality of life for thousands of people, because of one simple fact that you already know:

ENERGY
IS THE CURRENCY OF
LIFE.

I find it fascinating that everyone knows how important energy is, but hardly anyone knows how to improve their metabolism, which is where real energy comes from. Instead, they follow the latest energy fad, stand in line at the coffee shop, spend money on worthless "energy" drinks (hint: they're all useless), and because no amount of caffeine, herbs or magic fruit juice will truly improve metabolism, people never actually get the goods.

Perhaps you've followed one of the energy fads and been disappointed. Maybe you've tried a dozen products and none of them worked. Why read this book? Because, as my father was fond of saying, "It ain't bragging if you can prove it."

The Metabolic Makeover is not a product. It's a research-based, clinically documented program that produces dramatic improvements in the way your body creates, stores and uses energy. This book provides the details, but there is more than information here.

The Awareness Factor

As a university instructor, I was paid to provide information. I'm sure you noticed, however, that teachers who merely fulfilled that requirement didn't exactly light your fire. Think about it. Which teachers inspired you to change your point of view or change your life? They were the ones who provided more than information. They increased awareness; and awareness is personal.

Awareness is powerfully motivating, and usually leads to action. Awareness can change everything in the twinkling of an eye, and that's what I worked at with my students. Because in teaching people how their bodies work, the goal is not just to inform. The goal is to help them live long, healthy and joy-filled lives. You will see that I write like I teach, frequently asking questions in order to engage you and bring you to a better understanding of the magnificent human being that you are.

The Time Factor

Today of course, we have another hurdle. We're all so busy, and learning takes time. Thus, *The Metabolic Makeover* is designed to maximize learning efficiency. This is done with text, box-outs, diagrams, cartoons, pictures, and a summary at the end of each chapter. Biodialogs™ will help you understand the amazing and important cross-talk between different organs and systems that affects metabolic efficiency.

To create the dialog format, we're using this icon to represent the reader. This is where we sense that you, the reader, may need clarification on the topic being discussed.

This is my icon for replies.

This is Natalie's icon for replies.

We have spared no technique or technology in our quest to convey this important information to you. We're using social media and creating Metabolic Makeover webinars and seminars. Monthly updates are available at www.TheMetabolicMakeover. com, all because we believe that "if people knew better, they'd do better." This information is brand new, and when people GET it, they rapidly and easily improve the quality of their lives.

How will this improve my quality of life?

Imagine it's 25 years ago before GPS. You wanted to travel from Los Angeles to Denver, so you got something called a "map." For those born after the invention of GPS, this was an extremely large piece of paper with all the roads, cities and towns written on it. There were maps of every region of the US. Each map was folded about 65 times, and after use, could NEVER be refolded to the original shape.

But I digress. I want you to imagine that the map you bought for your trip to Denver was a discount map that was a reproduction of a map made in 1845. The recommended route took you south to the Sea of Cortez, then suggested rowing up the Colorado River 1,200 miles North to Denver. Estimated travel time: seven weeks.

Get the picture? With a current map showing the interstate highways, you could be in Denver in 15 hours. The important thing is to have the right map. Likewise, *The Metabolic Makeover* is the right map for your journey to greater energy and peak health.

How do I know *The Metabolic Makeover* is an accurate map?

Simple. Being a biochemist and a physician, Natalie and I are big on results that you can see, feel and measure. Most people start to see and feel improvements in a matter of days. These improvements are cumulative, and measurable in a matter of weeks. We're also big on documentation. *The Metabolic Makeover* includes more than 200 references to published biomedical literature.

To be successful, any health improvement effort has to be self-mo-

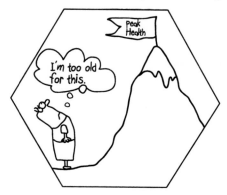

tivating. Every step has to build on the visible results of the previous step; otherwise, there's no energy, no juice, no enthusiasm, and you quit. Paddling up the Colorado River to Denver just gets too hard. And I'm sure you've noticed that aging makes giving up so much easier.

The Metabolic Makeover is results oriented and research based.

My science journey started in the 1950's at the start of the "space race." Like all 5th graders, I was given a government-mandated aptitude test that put me on the science and engineering track. This led to advanced studies in science and math, but more important a deep appreciation for the scientific method.

Decades later, as my career turned to the health sciences, I was dismayed at the lack of quality research in the emerging natural products arena. It seemed like everyone was content to just spin a story to sell the latest fad.

At the same time, my biomedical colleagues were more than happy to ignore botanical compounds in order to develop synthetic molecules that could be patented. By the 1990's, this had produced the worst of both worlds; a drug-only "health care" system that ignored prevention, and a natural products arena that could provide effective prevention but was mired in a swamp of confusion. Ultimately, I decided to retire from research and write books.

In 1997, I was living in Santa Barbara collecting checks from Random House for my first major book, The DHEA Breakthrough. The book was an international hit, and in conventional terms, I had it made.

THEN THE PHONE RANG.

You may have noticed that the universe appears to not like complacency. When you are satisfied with anything less than your highest and best, something comes along to shake things up. It can be misfortune, or something really good.

This phone call was about something really good; an opportunity to work on a global research project designed by a wealthy philanthropist named Bill Lee. I would have access to Bill Lee's vast agricultural resources (farms in every climate zone), an impressive medicinal plant library, and a state-of-the-art research facility staffed by experts in organic chemistry, botany, and molecular biology.

The project name was ECONET, and the goal was to build a bridge from the biomedical to the natural products side of the therapeutic fence. The ultimate goal was to rise above the hype with advanced technologies, including: genomics, proteomics, and proton nuclear magnetic resonance. The same analytical tools used by Big Pharma only instead of creating new-to-nature compounds with unknowable side effects, we'd be using plant-based compounds that have been part of the human experience since the dawn of creation.

Progress was swift. By 2003, the ECONET medicinal plant library contained over 10,000 plants and 150,000 fractions, all on a searchable database called Phytologix. With an automated microarray scanner, we could conduct 9,600 experiments in 24 hours. We could analyze the entire human genome in less than a week, combing through the Phytologix library for compounds that could reduce damage and enhance the body's inherent ability to repair and regenerate.

That year, I wrote *The Metabolic Plan*, in which I used this DNA-level understanding to map out a new way to look at and experience the aging process. The book was easy to understand, but more important it was actionable. When people followed the plan, they saw results.

FASTEN YOUR SEAT BELT.

In 2004, Tim Berners-Lee was knighted by the Queen of England for (among other things) pioneering the development of artificial Intelligence (AI). Modules were soon available that, placed in tandem with computational grids, could perform trillions of computations per second. That dramatically accelerated the discovery process worldwide, as prediction models replaced the trial-and-error methodology that had been the mainstay of science since Leonardo DaVinci.

By 2006, however, it was clear to me that many of my colleagues were getting lost in the sub-microscopic details. I have always believed that information is only truly valuable when it makes a difference in a person's life. And the difference I wanted to create was in heath care. All this science should have enabled us to create a revolution in health care, but where was the revolution?

The disconnect was profound. On the research side, the pace of change was absolutely blinding. On the clinical side, it was the same old, same old; what I call "drugs-for-bugs," or symptom-stomping. Most people still wait until something goes wrong, then take their body to the doctor just like they would take their car to a mechanic. In fact, people generally take better care of their cars, with an oil change every 3,000 miles, but completely neglect well-defined (and proven!) ways to prevent disease and degeneration in their own body.

The ECONET approach was to put more time and money into clinical research, and from 2007 to 2012, published 15 peer-reviewed studies demonstrating remarkable benefits obtained by human subjects using plant-based nutraceutical compounds.

If you build it, they will come.

We also started an education program to reach out to prevention-oriented physicians. The most common response to our doctor-only website was, "Finally...Someone's doing it right." This developed into a brain trust in which ECONET scientists shared the latest research and physicians shared their clinical experience with these compounds.

One of the clinical investigators in this brain trust was Dr. Natalie Kather. Board-certified in Family Practice and Anti-Aging medicine, Natalie had keen insights into what she called Metabolic Medicine. She needed a way to describe this new concept to her patients, and found that *The Metabolic Plan* was a big help. She reported that even if the patient only read the first three chapters, it shifted their awareness from expecting instant results to a willingness to begin a process of regeneration and renewal.

The collaborative experience of biochemist and physician worked on many levels. We are co-authors on this book, and as of June 9, 2012, life partners as well. Our synergy will be obvious as you travel through *The Metabolic Makeover*, because we are both passionate about learning. Her commentaries, called "Natalie Notes," will inform and inspire you.

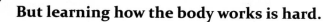

But learning how the body works is hard.

Learning is only difficult if you don't care or you have a bad teacher. I'm assuming that you care; otherwise, you wouldn't be reading this book. And I've made a career out of distilling complex information down to clear and accurate concepts. Natalie has pioneered what she calls the Partnership Health Care Model (see her Chapter 10) where the physician and patient work together to achieve optimal results. In both cases, we have had to refine and redefine the way we communicate.

Simple and True

You might have a safe deposit box in a bank where you keep your valuables. You are probably aware that the locking mechanism on that safe is incredibly complex, to say nothing about the three feet of cement and steel in which your box is encased. You don't care because you walk into the bank with what...?

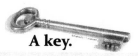

A key.

The Metabolic Makeover is based on clearly defined keys, and works as soon as you put these keys in the proper lock. It works fast, quite often in less than 30 days.

We're all familiar with reality-show makeovers, where people appear with great hair and fashion or return to a completely remodeled house. Unlike the reality shows, however, which slap on some makeup and a new outfit, we will be rebuilding and rejuvenating your body from the inside out.

Yes, you'll look better--guaranteed--but the real payoff will be in the way you feel: energized, enthusiastic, supple and strong. The miracle of the human body is all of us are constantly "renovating." The average adult replaces more than 300 billion cells every day.

That's a tremendous potential for regeneration and renewal, but most people waste this spectacular opportunity, simply because they do not know what to do. No one told them how to make vibrantly healthy cells, so they suffer with the process of degeneration, and their conventional doctor tells them to "learn to live with it."

Truth is, you can experience regeneration as early as your next meal. Whether your metabolism needs an overhaul or a minor tune-up; whether you're overweight and struggling with diabetes or an elite athlete, looking to break records, you need *The Metabolic Makeover*.

LET'S GET STARTED.

Chapter One

PARADOX

How long you...
Your children...
And your grandchildren live...
Depends increasingly...
On understanding the human genome.
  ~ *As The Future Catches You, Juan Enriquez*

Your genome is the sum total of your DNA. Some refer to it as "Command Central" because it contains all the information required by every cell in your body for your entire life. But it is not *centralized*, anywhere. A copy of your genome resides in nearly every cell. Since you have about 75 trillion cells, you might think that's a little redundant. But the magnificence of this system has produced every living thing, including bacteria, plants, animals and you.

Natalie and I believe that it is important for you to have a basic understanding of genomics (the activity of your genes) because that is what drives metabolism. Without this awareness, your body, and what happens to your body in this experience called life, will be a complete mystery to you.

Having this information, on the other hand, will enable you to *alter* or *improve* your metabolism, to produce greater and more consistent energy. You'll be able to burn fat and maintain your ideal weight. Most important, improving your metabolism will greatly reduce your risk for illness, disease and premature death.

Hopefully, you like to play Scrabble®. Because it's the best metaphor I can come up with to start this discussion. As you know, the entire Scrabble set contains 100 letter tiles, and you use these tiles to make words, using a maximum of seven letters in a turn. These 100 tiles can be arranged to create 178,691 possible words, which are listed in the Official Scrabble Players Dictionary. That's a lot of words.

So, Scrabble tiles form words from the 26 letters of the English alphabet. DNA creates proteins from only four chemical bases: (adenine, guanine, cytosine and thymine). Now here's the big difference that accounts for the multiplicity of organisms on this planet. The "words" that DNA can make are not limited to seven letters. In fact, the smallest human chromosome contains 50 million bases ("letters" in our scenario, here). The longest human chromosome contains about 250 million bases... and in your entire genome? About 3 billion bases. Imagine the number of "words" that nature can create from 3 billion "tiles." **Yes, mind officially blown.**

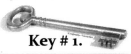

Key # 1.

The information required to build and maintain all living things is determined by the order, or sequence of the four DNA bases; similar to the way in which tiles in a Scrabble game are placed in a certain order to form words. Importantly, more than 99% of those bases are the same in all humans.

Can you see DNA under a microscope?

Not really. DNA is folded so tightly, it is generally considered sub-microscopic. Using an electron-scanning microscope, a chromosome is clearly visible, especially if it is stained. But remember that chromosomes (which organize genes into packages) can contain tens of thousands of genes.

Cells are microscopic, but if the DNA in a single human cell was unfolded and placed end to end, **it would be about six feet long.**

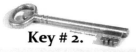
Key # 2.

This structure changes (evolves) very slowly over enormous spans of time. Painstaking genomic research tells us that the human genome has not changed much at all in the last 20,000 years. This is important, because during most of that time, we were Paleolithic hunters and gatherers. Which means that we are designed for:

- A highly varied natural foods diet
- Eating a number of small meals instead of the relatively massive intake of modern humans
- Periods of famine/hunger
- An extremely active lifestyle including a wide range of movements
- Episodic stress, as opposed to the chronic stress of the 21st century
- Sleep patterns that followed circadian rhythms

Then and Now

When I'm sitting in a 747, flying at 580 miles an hour, typing on my laptop and talking on the phone, I remind myself that I am a caveman dressed in a suit. My brain understands all this technology, but my body does not.

There is no way that our bodies could possibly have adapted to the astounding changes that have occurred in the last 5,000 years, let alone the last 100 years. We are in fact still tuned to the foods, conditions, activities and behaviors of the ancient past, but we live in a time warp where everything is different.

Our gastrointestinal tract is designed for grazing, whereas today we gorge. For two million years, whenever we became hungry, we simply picked something, ate it, and stopped eating as soon as our hunger was satisfied. Today, we postpone hunger to preset times called meals, whereupon we consume enormous amounts of food. Few of us stop when our hunger is gone; we eat until we're "full."

We can't go back to the Paleolithic times, and who would want to? The point is that awareness of our modern predicament, the fact that we are out of sync with our genes in many ways, opens the door to understanding how to vastly improve our quality of life.

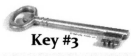

Key #3

The Paleolithic perspective is an important key in the quest for peak health whether you want to lose weight, maximize your lifespan, have more energy, enjoy deeper and more restoring sleep, improve your memory, boost your immunity, or all of the above. It is the foundation awareness that I will refer to in every chapter of this book, because it is the silent force encoded in your genes.

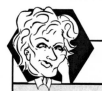

Why is this chapter entitled "Paradox?" Where's the paradox?

I was just about to get to that. I wanted you first to be grounded in the astounding complexity of the human genome, and its stability over millions of years. Now comes the paradox: it is also constantly changing.

I don't mean the genes *themselves* are changing, but the instructions that they are sending to the cells, tissues and organs can and do change. We are so used to thinking of DNA as a "blueprint," that it is hard to imagine a constantly changing, infinitely complex structure that is at all times aware of and responding to your physical, biochemical and emotional state.

SIT WITH THAT FOR A MOMENT.

Again, your genes don't change their chromosomal position, but their *activity* or *expression* can change. These are called epigenetic alterations. Think of a gene as a dimmer switch that can be on, off, or anywhere in between. Multiply that times 23,000 (the approximate number of genes in the human genome) and it is hard even for a scientist to grasp. If you ask a leading geneticist how many gene variations there are, he or she will say something rather cosmic, like "it's infinite."

It is hard to imagine a constantly changing, infinitely complex structure that is at all times aware of and responding to your physical, biochemical and emotional state.

Pop Quiz

There is an overall principle that has been observed regarding epigenetic alterations. It is the principle of efficiency. You see, your genome is concerned with one thing, and that is, choose one:

A. Your happiness
B. Your bank account
C. Your appearance
D. Your survival

Tick tock, tick tock...
Buzzer sound...

Answer: D: your survival.

And to optimize your chance of surviving (at least to child-bearing age), your genome is constantly adjusting to produce the most energy (required for growth and repair) while spending the least amount of energy; thus maximizing efficiency.

And of course the same is true for all living things, from fruit flies to redwood trees. It's like living in a magic house where every blind, curtain, door, vent and window was constantly adjusting to minimize energy expenditure while providing maximum comfort. Only the house that you live in is a million times more complex.

According to the principle of efficiency, fuel selection, utilization and storage are *primary* factors. And the two main fuels for human life are glucose (sugar) and fat.

Do you know any naturally thin people?

We all know people who can eat all they want and never gain an ounce. They never count calories, go on a diet, or have any concern about their weight. These are the *naturally thin people,* making up about 20% of the population in North America.

What's frustrating for the other 80%, is that naturally thin people are so darn *bubbly.* They tend to be optimists, and for good reason. They are naturally thin because, in metabolic terms, they won the DNA lottery. They inherited a metabolic advantage from their naturally thin parents: the ability to rapidly and easily burn fat.

Since burning fat provides slow and steady energy, naturally thin people tend to be athletic. Take any sport (other than football) and look at the players. There's a good portion of the 20%. Slow and steady energy also means they are not usually obsessed with food. Sometimes they forget to eat.

If you ARE a naturally thin person, this book is still valuable. It will help you get the most from your genetic gift, and importantly, help you maintain that advantage after age 40. That's right, aging is the great metabolic equalizer. Unless you learn how to control your metabolism, you may be one of those formerly naturally thin people who look in the mirror on their 50th birthday and wonder what happened.

If you ARE NOT a naturally thin person, this book is your key to a better life; greater and more consistent energy. It will improve your stamina and endurance, and the ability to maintain your ideal weight without having to go on a diet every two years.

In other words, *The Metabolic Makeover* is a program that can give any motivated person, the metabolic advantage of a naturally thin person. You can imagine the spectacular amount of money to be made by creating a drug that did that. Thus, the biomedical literature is filled with thousands of studies relating to energy metabolism, and every drug company I know has at least a few teams looking for the secret.

Truth is, it's not a secret. At least not any more. This vast amount of research shared in this book has uncovered a handful of enzymes and other signaling molecules that activate fat-burning pathways and confer remarkable metabolic advantages. But I'm willing to bet that it will never be a pill. It has to be a program. Turning on these pathways requires *action*, which is, of course, what this book is all about. Every chapter reveals another piece to the most exciting puzzle I can think of. Energy, after all is the currency of life.

Summary

1. In a very real sense, we are all out of synch with our genes. Technology changes rapidly, thus transforming every aspect of our lives. But the genes that control our cells haven't changed much at all in the last 20,000 years.

2. While genes don't change, their activity is constantly adjusting to the conditions of your life. These adjustments are called epigenetic changes.

3. Your genome runs on the principle of efficiency. Since creating energy from fat is slow compared to sugars/starches, your genome will reduce fat burning when your diet contains a lot of sugars and starches.

4. We should graze, not gorge. The gastrointestinal tract is designed for frequent, small meals.

Chapter Two

EVOLUTION/DEVOLUTION

*Perhaps our greatest distinction as a species is
our capacity, unique among animals, to make
counter-evolutionary choices.*

~ Guns, Germs & Steel: The Fates of Human Societies, Jared Diamond

You might be surprised to learn that Paleolithic men and women were healthier, stronger, and even taller than people in most modern societies. Sure, we have a higher overall life expectancy today, but if a hunter-gatherer made it to age 60, his or her chances of seeing 90 were just as good as yours. The point is that we now have the opportunity to surpass anything that has ever gone before as long as we don't forget where we came from.

Evolution

Evolution is not something that happened in the past. It's a process of refinement and growth that is never-ending. For millions of years, evolution occurred through natural selection. Genetic modifications resulted from hundreds of environmental events such as changes in the atmosphere set off by massive volcanic eruptions. These in turn produced climate changes that produced even more genetic modifications. The modifications that favored survival of a particular species were passed on, while modifications that reduced survival were obviously selected out...as organisms that fail to reproduce simply disappear.

This astounding process which—as you can understand—moves towards ever-increasing complexity, ultimately produced plants. Plants in the Middle East faced severe environmental challenges. In order to survive, they had to withstand harsh heat and dry summers. So how did this region become known as the "fertile crescent?"

In time, some plants survived by creating a seed that contained a large amount of starch encased in a hard shell. This seed was protected from the sun, yet could germinate at the first soaking rain. Even more important, the sprouting plant had enough fuel (starch) to survive while it sent roots deep enough to get more water. This was a monumental success for plants.

Then, about 12,000 years ago, humans migrating from the plains of Africa discovered this bonanza and it changed everything. Grains could be stored, and the hard shell could be ground with stone tools to release the starch for easy and fast digestion. Suddenly, there was no need to forage. Humans could survive on GRAIN.

Is it any wonder that bread became part of most religious rituals (i.e., "staff of life" and all that)? We cannot imagine how important grain was to these early humans. It saved them from starvation—and that was the situation until very recently when other foods became plentiful and affordable—and we invented refrigerators.

Devolution

1. Agriculture: the end of variety

As bands of hunter-gatherers started collecting, and then cultivating these early grains, it ushered in what is known as the agricultural revolution. While you were probably taught that this was an unmitigated blessing for humanity (allowing for permanent settlements that later became cities), anthropologists tell a different story.

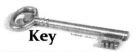
Key

Agriculture resulted in a dramatic reduction in food variety, leading to malnutrition and disease. Moreover, the dependence on one staple crop that was vulnerable to insects and drought (wheat, rice, corn), led to periodic famine, which in only a few generations, led to reduced lifespan. In the ensuing centuries, average adult height decreased by four inches. Evidence from skeletal remains suggests that these remarkable drawbacks persisted until about 5,000 years ago, meaning that agriculture dramatically reduced quality of life for over 7,000 years.

A return to hunting and gathering is clearly not an option for the seven billion people who now inhabit the earth. But we must understand the importance of a wide variety of plants and proteins.

2. Food Processing: disappearing nutrients

Refining and processing food removes critically important nutrients. Processing wheat into white flour, for example, eliminates 85% of the CoQ10, 90% of the vitamin E, and virtually all of the fiber. In all, 19 nutrients are reduced or destroyed. The fact that manufacturers then add thiamine, riboflavin and niacin back in and call the product "enriched," is a joke.

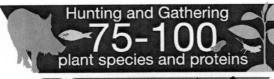

The Devolution Pyramid

Hunting and Gathering
75-100
plant species and proteins

Agricultural Era
Species shrank to staple crops

Refined & Processed Foods

Today's Typical American Diet
11 plant species

Vitamin A and beta carotene may survive some food processing, but they are very sensitive to oxidation and are protected only by the presence of vitamin E. When vitamin E is removed or destroyed (a common event), subsequent loss of vitamin A and beta carotene may be as high as 90%.[1] When beta carotene is added to margarine, 40% of the vitamin is destroyed while it is still being made.[2] By the time the product is shipped, stored and used, who knows if any of this nutrient is still available.

Virtually all essential nutrients are altered to some degree by food processing. Those that are most often depleted include: vitamins C, E, folic acid, B-6, thiamine, riboflavin, zinc, copper, magnesium, manganese, selenium and chromium.

Thus, by eating a highly-processed diet, you run the risk of being undernourished no matter how much food you eat. And no vitamin pill can make up for that. There are nutritional factors in whole natural foods that have not yet been identified. A new mineral was discovered in 1995. New flavonoids are identified every year.

> Eating a highly processed diet, you run the risk of being undernourished no matter how much food you eat.

The hunting-and-gathering diet was made up primarily of foods with a high-water content. The removal of water during processing improved shelf life and transportation, but also increased the number of calories in a bite of food. This is important because people generally regulate food intake by volume more than calories, so that over time, a processed food diet contributes directly to obesity.[3]

3. Sugar

O.K., so food processing in general is a problem because it reduces the number and amount of nutrients in the modern diet. But one type of processing towers above all others in terms of the damage and suffering it has caused.

This, of course, is the refining of cane and beet to create sugar.

Come on... Is sugar really poison?

Yes; slow-acting, but a poison nonetheless. And that's because all of the metabolic machinery that was created through millions of years of evolution was designed around the molecule known as glucose or blood sugar: $C_6H_{12}O_6$

For over 100,000 generations, glucose was delivered in complex "packages" known as starch. These starches or complex carbohydrates were found in a variety of roots, tubers, fruits and vegetables, so humans developed taste buds, a sensitive mechanism for the detection of starch. Because starch was so important as a fuel supply, the taste buds to detect its sweet taste covered two thirds of the tongue. And therein lies the problem.

For the hunter/gatherer, the predominance of sweet-taste sensors was a lifesaver, because it tipped them off to the presence of starch. Even so, paleoanthropologists estimate that hunters and gatherers were able to obtain only about 80 grams of carbohydrate per day. In fact, there was so little carbohydrate in our ancestor's diet that we evolved four ways of storing and making glucose:

Glucose is so important (especially for the brain) that we evolved four ways to store and generate this critical molecule.

1. Glucose is stored in the liver and muscles as glycogen
2. Glucose is stored in the blood as triglyceride
3. Glucose is stored in adipose tissue as fat
4. In a pinch, we can even convert protein into glucose

All of that machinery worked fine because glucose was derived from complex starches S L O W L Y through the process of digestion. Then, about 700 years ago, people figured out how to refine two particular starches down to a very simple substance known as sucrose or table sugar.

$$C_{12}H_{22}O_{11}$$

No longer were complex starches releasing glucose slowly into the bloodstream. Sucrose is digested by enzymes in saliva and raises blood glucose levels in a matter of seconds. As Europeans quickly discovered, one could eat sugar by the pound, and they did, knowing nothing about the disastrous consequences to their health.

The effect of this discovery was literally earth-shaking. Sugar produced an energy rush and a taste impact that fueled centuries of wars and colonial expansion. Sugar was the primary reason for the African slave trade, and vast areas of the Caribbean were destroyed to create sugar plantations.

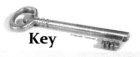
Key

Biochemically, sugar is also a disaster, because it raises glucose levels so fast and so high. Essentially, this throws a monkey-wrench into the body's intricate metabolic machinery. Everyone knows that a spike in blood sugar causes problems for the pancreas, and I'll describe that spiral of destruction in a bit. But even before stressing the pancreas, liver and kidneys, elevated blood sugar wreaks havoc in the human body. Not surprisingly, the immediate damage occurs in the cells lining the blood vessels that have direct contact with glucose. This is one of the initial causes of atherosclerosis and cardiovascular disease.[4]

Altered blood sugar metabolism contributes directly to a raft of diseases including obesity, diabetes (now called diabesity) and also osteoporosis, cancer, kidney disease, vision loss and blindness. Since elevated blood glucose is so dangerous, the body responds by secreting insulin, the hormone responsible for taking glucose out of the blood stream and into the cells.

But remember, this mechanism was designed for slowly digesting starches. The massive increase in glucose resulting from modern sugar consumption overwhelms the body's ability to maintain this critical balance, producing a rollercoaster of energy followed by fatigue. When blood glucose and insulin levels are high, brain biochemistry may be altered, producing mood swings and confusion. When blood glucose levels drop, symptoms of tiredness, anxiety, depression, irritability, disorientation and headache are all intensified.[5]

The issue here is metabolic stress. Biochemically, the body is simply not equipped for intake of pure glucose—and although it will adapt and function—the pancreas, liver, adrenals, kidneys, blood vessels and heart will be strained in the process.

Dr. Sheldon Reiser, former head of the carbohydrate lab at the USDA's Human Nutrition Institute, points out that two early signs of diabetes develop when people consume excess sugar: high insulin and high glucose levels. Dr. Reiser recommended drastic reduction of refined sugar intake, suggesting that "a national campaign be launched to inform the populace of the hazards of excessive sugar consumption."[6] That was in 1978, when the per capita intake of sugar was about 12 tsp. per day. Nothing was done. Twenty years later, a coalition of health agencies and public health experts petitioned the USDA to review escalating sugar consumption, citing medical evidence that it posed a national public health threat. Nothing was done.

Today, the average American consumes about 24 teaspoons of sugar (e.g., table sugar, dextrose, corn syrup, etc.) per day, amounting to nearly 150 pounds of sugar per person each year.[8] We're creating problems that evolution cannot possibly solve.

Then and Now

THEN (for 2 million years)

Complex carbohydrates that digest slowly, provided time-released energy over the course of many hours. Blood sugar balance was maintained by a high fiber, high protein diet and the activities of daily life.

Natalie note

The medical view of devolution

The life-shortening effect of diabetes is approximately 13 years. Because of this, the overall life-expectancy of Americans is expected to decline as the obesity, type 2 diabetes, kidney and liver disease epidemic takes its toll on generations X, Y and Z. We physicians are already having to manage these diseases in teenagers and young adults, and sometimes children; conditions that 20 years ago were only seen in adult and older adult medicine. Experts now warn that the present generation may be the first in history to have a **shorter life span than their parents.**[9]

We no longer call type 2 diabetes "adult onset diabetes," since it is now more common in younger populations. Nonalcoholic steatohepatitis (NASH) was named to differentiate it from the previously more common liver disease caused by excess alcohol consumption. NASH is caused by the accumulation of fat in the liver, often resulting from high consumption of soft drinks, saturated fat, and junk food. When I see a 16-year-old with liver disease, I want to cry, because the prognosis is bleak. Unless drastic measures are taken to reduce fat and sugar intake, this young person will face a lifetime of chronic disease.

The US Department of Health and Human Services has issued guidelines advising physicians to screen 11-year-olds for high cholesterol. I am also told to be watchful for childhood hypertension (high blood pressure), often due to other disease states like kidney disease. And all of this; the increasing incidence of high cholesterol, fatty liver, diabetes and hypertension is tied to obesity, caused by 21st century devolution.[10]

Milestones to Madness

1250 AD: Trade routes established to India and China, bringing refined sugar to Europe

1500 AD: Europeans "discover" land in the Caribbean suitable for growing cane. Slave trade begins to produce enough sugar to supply insatiable worldwide demand. From 1500 to 1865, it is estimated that more than 10 million Africans were enslaved to work on sugar, coffee, cocoa and cotton plantations.

1851: Jacob Fussell in Baltimore established the first large-scale commercial ice cream plant

1899: First bottle of Coca Cola

1900: Average North American sugar consumption per person is 1 pound per year

1920: Harry Burt invented the Good Humor Ice Cream Bar

1921: Wonder Bread

1930: Hostess Twinkie

1934: The first Eskimo Pie chocolate covered ice cream bar on a stick

1950: Dunkin' Donuts; "America's favorite all-day, everyday stop for coffee and baked goods."

1950s Kellogg's Frosted Flakes® and Tony the Tiger®

1957: High fructose corn syrup

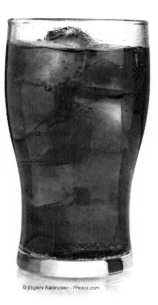
© Evgeny Karandaev - Photos.com

By the end of the 1950s, there were 29 Krispy Kreme shops in 12 states, each having the capacity to produce 500 DOZEN doughnuts per hour via high-speed doughnut-making machines

1960: Reuben Mattus launches Häagen-Dazs

1989: Red Bull (now making 4 billion cans a year)

2010: Average North American sugar consumption, per person is **150 pounds per year!**

You are starting to see the incredible disconnect between the diet that we were designed for and the diet that we presently consume. Acquiring calories is now nearly effortless, but our bodies are still hard wired to store every calorie that enters our mouth. This is the ancient blueprint that is preparing for a possible famine. Your DNA simply doesn't know that in your kitchen is a refrigerator and pantry bursting with calories.

In the next chapter we'll look at a particular kind of calorie.

Summary

1. The "agricultural revolution" was a mixed blessing.

2. Humans have been collecting and cultivating grain for only about 12,000 years. In evolutionary terms, that is the blink of an eye.

3. Devolution occurs when conditions are created which reduce a species' survivability. Three devolutionary forces have been agriculture, food processing and the refining of sugar.

Endnotes

1   De Ritter E. Stability characteristics of vitamins in processed foods. Food Technol, 1976. 30:48-54.

2   Marusich W, De Ritter E, Bauernfeind JC. Provitamin A activity and stability of beta carotene in margarine. J Am Oil Chem Soc, 1959. 34:217.

3   Rolls BJ. The relationship between dietary energy density and energy intake. Physiol Behav, 2009. 97(5):609-615.

4   Piga R, Naito Y, Kokura S, Handa O, Yoshikawa T. Short-term high glucose exposure induces monocyte-endothelial cells adhesion and transmigration by increasing VCAM-1 and MCP-1 expression in human aortic endothelial cells. Atherosclerosis, 2007. 193:328-334.

5   Salzer HM. Relative hypoglycemia as a cause of neuropsychiatric illness. J National Med Assoc, 1966. 58:12.

6   Reiser S, Szepesi B. SCOGS report on the health aspects of sucrose consumption. Am J Clin Nutr, 1978. Jan;31(1):9-11.

7   Reiser S, Szepesi B. SCOGS report on the health aspects of sucrose consumption. Am J Clin Nutr, 1978. Jan;31(1):9-11.

8   Burley VJ. Sugar consumption and human cancer in sites other than the digestive tract. Eur J Cancer Prev., 1998. Aug;7(4):253-77.

9   Olshansky SJ, Passaro DJ, Hershow RC, Layden J, Carnes BA, Brody J, Hayflick L, Butler RN, Allison DB, Ludwig DS. A potential decline in life expectancy in the United States in the 21st century. N Engl J Med., 2005 Mar 17; 352(11):1138-45.

10 Hansen ML, Gunn PW, Kaelber DC. Underdiagnosis of Hypertension in Children and Adolescents JAMA. 2007; 298(8):874-879. doi:10.1001/jama.298.8.874.

Chapter Three

THE CARB CONVERSATION

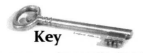
Key

All carbohydrates are converted to glucose. And whether this helps you (by providing energy) or harms you, all depends on the

AMOUNT of carbohydrate
and the *SPEED*
by which it enters the blood stream.

A metabolic emergency is created every time glucose levels overwhelm the body's control mechanisms that were designed through millions of years of natural selection. While this metabolic stress often leads to Type 2 diabetes, it is important to understand that significant damage is done long before that disease occurs.

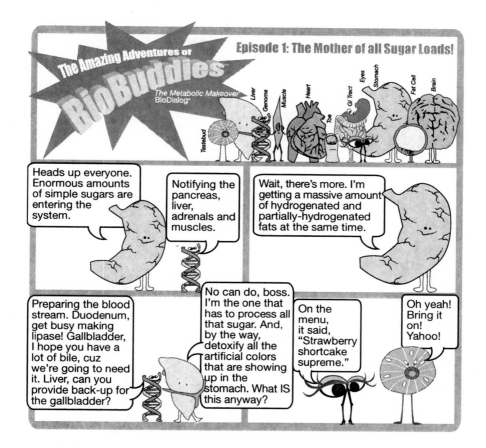

Carbohydrate 101

I've read hundreds of scientific studies that used the term carbohydrate without making the distinction between unprocessed, complex foods like whole grains and refined/processed carbs, like cakes, cookies and doughnuts. This demonstrates the utter confusion that exists in this arena, even at the scientific level.

In truth, there are three major factors that necessitate precision when using the term carbohydrate. That is because other dietary factors (often in the same food) affect the impact of carbohydrate on metabolic balance.

The first is fiber. Fiber slows down carbohydrate digestion and glucose delivery. To a lesser degree, so do fats and protein. It is therefore reasonable to say that whole foods (including whole grains, vegetables and fruit) are metabolically superior to refined grains and processed fruits and vegetables. An apple is far better for you than a glass of apple juice. Strawberries are better than a Fruit Roll-Up®. Brown rice is better than white rice (although quinoa provides even more fiber and less carbs); whole barley is better than refined "pearl" barley; old-fashioned, steel-cut oats are better than instant oatmeal; whole peas (fresh or frozen) are better than flavored, dried "snack" peas. Cranberries are better than Craisins®.

O.K. We get it

Just one more example: In 2010, dried blueberries started showing up everywhere, with one leading brand extolling the goodness of "whole dried blueberries picked at the height of freshness." You had to read the label carefully to learn that they were "infused" with sugar; lots of sugar, 28 grams of sugar per 1/3 cup serving. That's nearly six times the sugar content of fresh blueberries.

"Strawberry Splash Fruit Gushers have only a trivial amount of strawberries (from concentrate), presumably for the purpose of marketing. The product contains highly-processed ingredients never before present in the food supply, including 7 variants of sugar and partially-hydrogenated fat."

~ DAVID S. LUDWIG, MD, PHD. TECHNOLOGY, DIET, & THE
BURDEN OF CHRONIC DISEASE. JOURNAL OF THE AMERICAN
MEDICAL ASSOCIATION, APRIL 6, 2011 – VOL 305, NO.13.

Keeping Score

Today, you can get into the minute details of carbohydrate metabolism thanks to myriad websites, books and articles listing the glycemic index (GI) of hundreds of foods. This is a measure of how rapidly a certain food will raise blood-sugar levels, relative to pure glucose. Glucose is given a value of 100, so presumably, a food with a GI of 50 would raise blood sugar at half the rate of pure glucose.

Over the last 20 years, debate has raged over the relevance and value of GI lists. Glycemic index weight loss diets have been launched, along with guidelines for diabetics and cancer patients, and pro/con arguments have appeared in most nutrition and metabolism journals.

Here is Natalie's take on the Glycemic Index.

Natalie note The glycemic index helped me understand that there is very little difference between a cookie and a slice of bread, since both raise blood sugar at about the same rate. I have used these concepts to help my patients make better food choices, but I advise against basing one's diet on the glycemic index tables.

First of all, no one eats just one food at a meal, so the GI of a complex meal is impossible to determine. Besides, eating should be enjoyable, and should not require the calculator function of your smartphone.

In addition, GI values can vary according to the ripeness of the food, the way it is cooked, and even its temperature. Cold potato salad has a much lower GI than a baked potato. And most important, the GI is affected by the amount consumed. GI val-

35

ues are determined based on a serving that provides 50 grams of carbohydrate. If you just look at the chart, carrots are listed as a high GI food, but to get 50 grams of carbohydrate, you'd have to eat more than 3 cups of carrots. All at once. And even then, the GI would depend on how fast you ate these carrots, how well they were chewed, and—this is key—your muscle-to-fat ratio.

You see the problem. We'd like to think that the glycemic index is the key to losing weight, managing your blood sugar, and living a long, happy life, but it is only useful as a general guide. Does anyone need to be told that they should avoid high GI foods like white bread, sweetened breakfast cereals, fruit juice, soft drinks, cakes, cookies and candy?

Oh, I know plenty of people who do not have that information.

O.K. an updated international GI list is available at: **http://www.mendosa.com/gilists.htm.** What's more, this excellent resource also provides data on glycemic load (GL) which I find more useful. Glycemic load takes into account the serving size and the available carbohydrate. Available carbohydrate (also known as net carbs) includes the starch and sugar, minus the fiber. Glycemic load data corrects a number of errors found in the GI tables, such as the listing of watermelon and carrots as high GI foods, when both have low glycemic load values.

The Metabolic Makeover Bottom-Line Carb Guidelines

1. Avoid refined sugar products like the plague that they, in fact, are.

2. Avoid soft drinks, including the biggest health scam ever launched: "diet" soft drinks.

3. Re-tune your taste buds. It is important to enjoy your food, but food chemists have invented compounds that trick you into eating more than you need. They're not kidding when they say, "Bet you can't eat just one."

   As you increase your intake of unprocessed whole natural foods, especially raw vegetables and legumes, you will be surprised at how fast your taste receptors become sensitive to the more subtle but no less enjoyable flavors and textures.

4. Never eat "unopposed carbs." Try to consume a high-fiber protein before or with carbohydrates. Our motto: never be more than an arm's distance from a handful of almonds (120 calories, 5g protein, 3g fiber and 2 (that's right, TWO!)g net carbs). Example: concord grapes have a GI of 59 (fairly high). A handful of concord grapes and a handful of almonds: 20.[1]

   Remember that fiber, fat and protein all moderate the glycemic impact of carbs, and this is particularly true of the amino acid, leucine.[2] High leucine foods include seeds, nuts, beans, beef and fish.

Why are you spending so much time talking about carbs?

Because life is fundamentally about how energy is obtained, stored, and used. And for animals, including you and me, the amazingly complex machinery and biochemistry is all built around glucose, obtained from carbohydrates.

I started to GET this in the 4th grade, when my teacher put a chart like this on the wall:

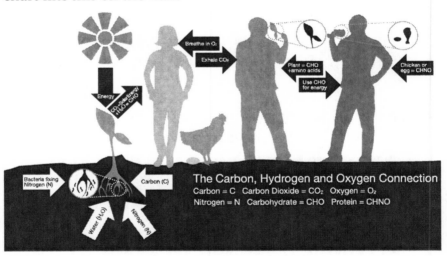

The Carbon, Hydrogen and Oxygen Connection
Carbon = C   Carbon Dioxide = CO_2 Oxygen = O_2
Nitrogen = N   Carbohydrate = CHO   Protein = CHNO

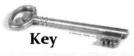

Key

I was mesmerized by that chart because it awakened an ancient memory encoded in my DNA that connects all living things through carbon, hydrogen and oxygen. Carb-O_2-hydrate.

But again, I want to describe how this connection has been strained.

Then and Now

To obtain a day's worth of carbohydrate— about 80 grams— from roots, tubers and berries, your ancestors had to forage about 4 hours. At the same time, they used up a large number of calories foraging, which resulted in the fact that there were no overweight hunters and gatherers.

Calculation # 1

Calories burned to acquire 80 grams carbohydrate by a hunter/gatherer = **about 250.**

With constant access to high-GI foods like potatoes and pasta, along with baked goods, candies, soft drinks, breakfast cereals, granola bars, sweets and desserts, it is not unusual for North Americans to consume 500 grams of carbohydrates every day. Calories burned to obtain 500 grams carbohydrates - 40 (opening the refrigerator or the pantry, driving to the cupcake shop).

Calculation # 2

One gram of carbohydrate provides 4 calories of energy. So the hunting/gathering diet provided about **320 calories from carbs.**

The modern diet, by contrast, provides almost **2,000 carb calories.** And to complete the picture + add roughly 90 grams of protein x 4 calories per gram = **360** + a whopping 100 grams of fat x 9 calories per gram = **900 calories.** For a total of ....

DRUM ROLL ...

3,260 calories per day! Try staying fit on that!

Your genome runs on the principle of ... Anyone? Anyone?

Remember that your genome is constantly monitoring your situation and behavior, looking for the most efficient way to run your body. To convert carbs to sugar and sugar to energy is simple and fast. To burn fat—that is, to move fat from your thighs to your liver or muscle to create energy—is metabolically very "expensive."

First, since the fat has to travel through the blood stream, it has to be made water-soluble; a process called hydrolysis. That requires a two-step enzyme process. The resulting fatty acids are then carried by transport proteins to the target tissue (e.g., liver, muscle, heart).

But that's just the beginning. Other transport proteins are required to get the fatty acid into the target cell. Then, a number of enzymes, including carnitine and carnitine palmitoyl tranferase [CPT-1] are required to transport the fatty acid across the outer and inner mitochondrial membrane. The resulting molecule, fatty-acyl carnitine, reacts with coenzyme A to produce acetyl-CoA, and THAT is the fuel that enters the Krebs Cycle to produce energy. **W h e w !**

Compare that to carbohydrate metabolism. Ready? Carbohydrate is reduced to glucose by amylase. This starts in your mouth before you even swallow the cookie/bagel/candy. Glucose is already water soluble, so transport is swift. Glucose is escorted into the cell by insulin, converted to pyruvate and then AcetylCoA. **Done!**

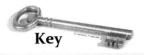

Key

Burning fat is difficult and metabolically "expensive." Burning sugar is fast and easy. Thus, when faced with an abundance of sugar, the human genome adjusts to down-regulate fat-burning machinery. This is the story of the 20th century, and the reason why 65% of adults in North America are overweight and tired.

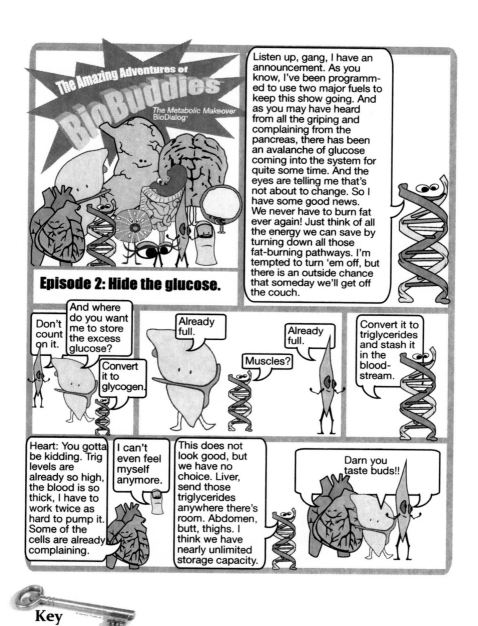

Key

So, you now understand that the glycemic index and glycemic load numbers not only reflect the impact of the food on glucose balance, but also the degree to which that food suppresses the body's ability to burn fat.

Let me put this another way. My first nutrition instructor called sugar and other refined carbs "empty calories;" implying that the only problem was that they replaced more nutritious foods. We now know that refined carbs set off a chain-reaction of damage that includes preventing the body from burning fat.

A little history

Importantly, this adaptation to a high-carb diet started right after WWII. You see, scientists started using nitrates and phosphates to make explosives in WWI. It was then discovered that these same compounds could make plants grow in virtually any soil; even in the dust-bowl states and the Canadian prairies. So by the end of WWII, production of wheat and corn was skyrocketing in North America from coast to coast.

The resulting surplus would have crashed the commodity markets if the US and Canadian governments had not embarked upon a historic intervention, purchasing more than 100 million bushels of wheat. Canada stored their surplus in gigantic grain elevators that still dot the prairie provinces. The US stashed the wheat in retired battleships and cargo ships, anchored in the Hudson River. I find it ironic that I grew up looking at what was called the "mothball fleet:" 189 massive ships filled with wheat. And the other major fleet (100 additional ships) was moored in Olympia WA, where I now reside.

Even with government intervention, you could still buy a bushel of wheat in 1950 for less than a dollar, meaning that a box of breakfast cereal could be made for about 10¢. With a profit margin like that, the breakfast cereal explosion was born, complete with cartoon characters advertising directly to children on the new invention called television.

It took less than a decade for advertisers to alter the course of human history, starting with breakfast, but then extending to lunch, dinner and an endless variety of snacks. Wonder Bread ("Helps Build Strong Bodies 12 Ways") was advertised by Howdy Doody and Buffalo Bob.[4]

Trucks also started coming through my neighborhood. The "bread man" handed out samples of cakes, cookies and other sugary treats to all the mothers and their eager kids. Bread, rolls, muffins, coffeecake, pies, cupcakes, brownies, croissants, cookies, "crullers" and bear claws. Then it was Ring Dings, Devil Dogs, Sara Lee, Drakes Cakes, Hostess Twinkies, Animal Crackers, Pepperidge Farm, TastyKakes, Dolly Madison, Little Debbie, Famous Amos and the Pillsbury Doughboy. My sister collected Betty Crocker coupons at home and baked Duncan Hines cakes at school, doing her part to empty those cargo ships.

The down-regulation of fat-burning metabolic pathways was an epigenetic adaptation at first. But it was then passed on, so that every generation after 1945 has become fatter and more diabetic.

A Little Ancient History

Students would often ask me why humans did not simply evolve ways to manage excess glucose. After all, we don't seem to have a problem with large amounts of protein, and even large amounts of fat do not set off a metabolic alarm until we reach the obese state.

The answer has to do with the dietary forces that shaped our current digestive system. Think Paleolithic.

* There were extended periods of time when we ate enormous amounts of protein. We're talking wooly mammoth, buffalo, rhinoceros, deer, elk and other large mammals that are now extinct.

* There were also extended periods of time when we ate large amounts of fat. Think long, hard winters. The traditional Eskimo diet was—until recently—roughly 65% fat.

Now, was there ever a time—during literally millions of years—that humans ate enormous amounts of refined carbohydrates?

No. Humans could not possibly evolve mechanisms to handle something that did not occur. The dilemma we face today is that our technology (the ability to create unlimited amounts of sugar) has outstripped our biology.

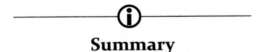

Summary

1. Through the process of digestion, all carbohydrates are converted to the simple sugar known as glucose.

2. Whole, natural foods contain a mixture of carbohydrate, fat, protein and fiber. This combination slows delivery of glucose into the bloodstream.

3. Food processing (destroying the balance of carb, fat, protein and fiber) speeds delivery of glucose into the bloodstream.

4. The glycemic index is a measure of the speed by which a food raises blood glucose levels. It is useful as a general guideline, but cannot accurately determine the metabolic effect of a complex meal.

5. Carbohydrates are not the enemy. Processed, sweetened, chemicalized, low-fiber carbs are. Think like a hunter/gatherer. There are no bagel trees or spaghetti bushes.

Endnotes

1   De Natale C, Annuzzi G, Bozzetto L, et al. Effects of a Plant-Based High-Carbohydrate/High-Fiber Diet Versus High–Monounsaturated Fat/Low-Carbohydrate Diet on Postprandial Lipids in Type 2 Diabetic Patients. Diabetes Care, December 2009 vol. 32 no. 12 2168-2173

2   Kalogeropoulou D, Lafave L, Schweim K, Gannon MC, Nuttall FQ. Leucine, when ingested with glucose, synergistically stimulates insulin secretion and lowers blood glucose. Metabolism. 2008 Dec;57(12):1747-52.

3   at least a dozen people in North America are each recorded to weigh more than 1,000 pounds

4   Go here to see the actual ad. http://www.youtube.com/watch?v=hh-D_13mbJQY&feature=results_main&playnext=1&list=PL45342941ABC-91FAE

Chapter Four

THE TRIPLE WHAMMY

We've explained how a high-carb diet overwhelms the body's glucose balancing mechanism. Basically, it's too much fuel entering the system too fast. In an effort to handle the glucose load, the liver converts as much as possible to glycogen.

Picture this: blood glucose levels rising. Genome tells the liver to handle it, and then an astounding process occurs. The liver creates a protein core, and then starts arranging glucose molecules around that core, creating a physical structure that resembles a sphere. Each molecule of glycogen can contain – ready? 20,000 glucose units. When each glycogen molecule is completed, the liver looks for a place to put it. Since the liver itself has limited storage space, it relies on the muscles to hold most of this amazing backup energy source.

NOTE: The creation and transport of glycogen happens in a matter of seconds. It occurs in your body every day, multiple times a day. Then, later on, your muscles can literally peel off as many glucose units as they need in order to perform whatever exercise or movement you require.

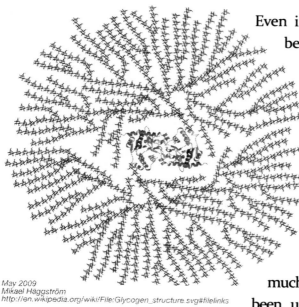

Even in 2 D, glycogen is a beautiful thing. Between meals (or when you exercise) glycogen is easily and rapidly converted back to glucose. But here's another Paleolithic rub: the amount of glycogen the muscles can hold depends on how much those muscles have been used. Our Paleolithic ancestors were incredibly active, and most of us are not. Thus, the modern era not only brought us an avalanche of glucose, but a dramatic reduction in our ability to store it as glycogen.

As you might guess, exercise produces incredibly beneficial changes in the glycogen storage cycle. Exercise activates genes which stimulate glycogen storage capacity, which gives you more available energy and greater stamina. This is called the Training Effect, making exercise easier and more enjoyable.

It also means that more dietary carbohydrates are converted to energy and less to fat. With consistent exercise, liver storage of glycogen also increases, as does the speed at which this glycogen is made available to the body. An active person will have up to 20 times the amount of stored glycogen as a sedentary person of equal weight ... and a trained athlete can more than double that! In Chapter 9, you will learn which type of exercise has the greatest effect on the glycogen/energy/stamina cycle.

> The modern era not only brought us an avalanche of glucose, but a dramatic reduction in our ability to store it as glycogen.

Whammy # 1: Insulin Resistance

Now, what happens to the more than 65% of North American adults who are not physically fit? Remember that insulin is signaling the cells to take up glucose, but as the storage sites (liver and muscle) fill up with glycogen, those cells become resistant to the insulin signal, and glucose remains in the blood.

Whammy # 2: Elevated Glucose

Since excess glucose is toxic, the pancreas furiously pumps out more insulin, which only makes the cells more resistant. Eventually, the liver (yes, the liver again) manages to convert excess glucose to two types of fat. The first is called triglyceride, a combination of glucose (glycerol) and fat that gets stored in the bloodstream. As blood levels rise, these triglycerides are dispatched to the thighs, abdomen, arms, legs and buttocks, where they add to adipose tissue.

NOTE: As you probably realize, this ability to store energy in the bloodstream, liver, muscles and adipose tissue was – for 2 million years, the key to our survival. But here we are in the 21st century, with no predators to flee from, no famines to deal with, an overabundance of calories and a sedentary lifestyle: clearly, a recipe for disaster.

Triglycerides are a waxy substance floating in the blood. High levels of triglycerides greatly increase the viscosity (thickness) of the blood and are thus a major risk factor for cardiovascular disease. When people have high levels, it can even make their blood look creamy. I once had a patient whose triglycerides were so high that when we spun the test tube of his blood in a centrifuge, it looked like a white candle. It was as if we could stick a wick in it and light it. And this fellow's heart was trying to pump that sludge through 50,000 miles of blood vessels to about 75 trillion cells.

People often do not realize that when they eat bread, cookies, cake, pasta and potatoes they are creating more triglycerides and more wax in their bloodstream. I want my patients to keep trigs under 100 mg/dL. To put this into perspective, an athlete will typically have trigs in the 30 to 60 range. Why? Because they are, on a daily basis, using trigs to fuel exercise.

IT GETS WORSE

Are you starting to see the relationship between muscle and fat? In an active person, muscle burns fat. In a sedentary person, fat damages muscle. That's because adipose (fat) tissue doesn't just sit there. It secretes inflammatory proteins called adipokines, which damage nearby muscle.

> An active person will have up to 20 times the amount of stored glycogen as a sedentary person of equal weight ... and a trained athlete can more than double that!

When muscle is damaged, its ability to burn fat declines, which accelerates the accumulation of fat. As the adipose cells fill up, they start to unload excess fat into adjacent muscle, which lowers the metabolic efficiency of muscle even further.

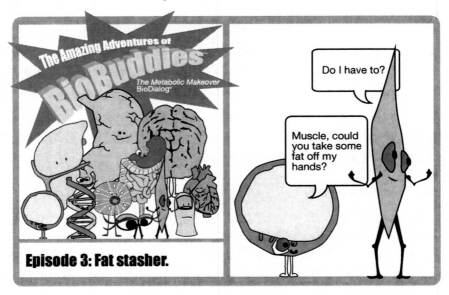

Whammy # 3: Inflammation

Excess glucose, meanwhile, causes inflammation wherever it goes. In the blood stream, inflammation begins the process of atherosclerosis. In the brain, inflammation creates the damage leading to dementia. Inflammation in the internal organs compromises kidney and liver function, and inflammation is involved in all three stages of cancer: initiation, progression and metastasis.

Levels of insulin remain high as the pancreas continues its effort to drive glucose into tissues that have no room or metabolic need for that fuel. And high-insulin levels in turn, contribute to the cycle of destruction by elevating blood pressure, damaging blood vessels and accelerating tumor growth.

The Insulin Cancer Connection

As a physician, I am well aware that high serum insulin is a major risk factor for cardiovascular disease and vision loss. But as Stephen and I looked into this further, we found that excess insulin also increases the risk for cancer. Researchers have found that Type 2 diabetic patients receiving insulin therapy have twice the risk of colorectal cancer compared to those not receiving insulin therapy.[1] What's more, new research suggests that elevated insulin increases cancer risk long before the diabetic state.[2]

Choices.

The combination of insulin resistance, elevated glucose and inflammation wreaks havoc throughout the body. Insulin resistance not only prevents glucose from entering muscle cells, it also prevents the uptake of amino acids. Thus, someone with insulin resistance will have a hard time building or even maintaining their muscle mass. And going to their conventional doctor, they are likely to hear:

> "Mr. Jones, you've gained 10 pounds in the last year, and your blood pressure, cholesterol and fasting blood glucose numbers are all up. This is a worrisome trend, and if you want to avoid diabetes, you're going to have to exercise more and lose weight."

Now, that's an accurate statement, but bad advice.

Huh?

You see, when Mr. Jones goes to the gym, here's what happens. His insulin resistance has created a situation where his ability to convert fuel to energy is severely impaired. He has already lost muscle strength and probably muscle size. Because of his high-carb diet, his body has stopped making fat-burning enzymes. Thus, with the exercise tolerance of a garden slug, he signs up for an aerobics class. This will not turn out well.

By the end of the 10 minute warm-up, he has already decided never to try that again. The fact that other people are invigorated and happy is a complete mystery to him. He blames himself, and subconsciously surrenders to the downward spiral of Metabolic Syndrome, the constellation of symptoms including elevated blood sugar, blood pressure, cholesterol, triglycerides and body fat.

An alternate end to this story.

If his doctor was skilled in metabolic medicine, Mr. Jones would have received different advice.

This is the dialog Natalie would have had with Mr. Jones:

Natalie:

"Mr. Jones, you've gained 10 pounds in the last year, and your blood pressure, cholesterol and fasting blood glucose numbers are all up. This is a worrisome trend, but it's all reversible. You're at a crossroads. If you do nothing, by next year, I'll have to write you a handful of prescriptions: one or two for your

blood pressure, one for your cholesterol, and at least two for your blood sugar.

But I have to inform you that those drugs are only designed to deal with your symptoms. They won't do much at all to correct the underlying cause of your problem. In fact, they often work against each other, with drugs prescribed for blood pressure adversely affecting your blood sugar, forcing me to add another drug – a TZD, some of which have already been withdrawn from the market because of serious adverse effects on the heart & liver.

Mr. Jones:
But I thought part of my problem was impaired liver function.

Natalie:
Exactly, and most pharmaceutical drugs stress the liver; some more than others. And look at this: new research shows that TZD's actually stimulate the formation of new fat cells. So they contribute directly to the worst kind of weight gain.[3]

Mr Jones:
But I'm trying to lose weight!

Natalie:
Which will be next to impossible on these drugs because they reduce exercise tolerance. You'll be lucky to get up a flight of stairs without feeling tired. You'll gain weight, have trouble sleeping, be at increased risk for congestive heart failure, liver disease and some types of cancer. But your blood pressure, blood sugar and cholesterol will all be in the normal range.

Mr. Jones:
Oh for crying out loud! You said I'm at a crossroads. What's the other choice?

Natalie:

It's called The Metabolic Makeover; a program designed to get you out of this precarious situation. You see, Mr. Jones, you do not have a statin, TZD, atenolol, biguanide, diuretic or lisinopril deficiency. You're in a metabolic tail-spin and time is not on your side. All of these issues become harder to correct as we age.

Mr Jones:

O.K. Where do I start?

START HERE

Mr. Jones' problem— and the challenge faced by more than 150 million people in North America—is that Metabolic Syndrome is a very complex issue. And conventional medicine is terrible with complex disorders. They like to have one specific target so they can develop a drug to crush it. So the conventional response to Metabolic Syndrome is NOT to understand the complex interplay of fundamental causes, but to prescribe a drug for each of the eventual results; what Natalie calls "symptom-stomping." She adds:

"The drug-only treatment of Metabolic Syndrome is like plastering the cracks in the wall of a house that is sliding down a hill. The real problem is the foundation."

First thing's first;

Astute readers are already saying, "Duh! Mr. Jones has to stop eating so many carbs." And you're right. By reducing the amount of glucose entering the system, he can dramatically reduce his metabolic stress. For many people, however, that's easier said than done.

What's so hard? Can't he just make better food choices?

Theoretically, yes. But if that were easy, wouldn't everyone have already done this? Sweets are our comfort foods, our reward foods, and they trigger changes in brain chemistry that strongly affect our moods. Carbohydrate addiction is a real phenomena, stemming from biochemical, social and evolutionary forces. Stephen and I attended a seminar recently on Diabetes Research. There were bowls of candy at every table. And they had to be refilled every day.

In every language, practically every endearing term refers to sweetness. Think about it.

Sweetheart *Cupcake* *Sugar* *Honey* *Cutie Pie*

The USDA started begging Americans to eat at least 5 daily servings of fruits and vegetables back in 1990, when half of the adults in the US were overweight or obese. Today, fully two thirds of Americans are overweight or obese. Apparently, the "Eat Five to Stay Alive" USDA slogan was drowned out by scores of opposing slogans like:

> *"Nothin says lovin like something from the oven. And Pillsbury says it best."*

> *"Arby's. It's Good Mood Food!"*

> *"You deserve a break today."*

"Coke. It's the real thing."

"It takes two hands to hold a Whopper."

"America Runs On Dunkin."

"Hardee's. Come on Home."

"Love Bacon? Marry It." (Jack in the Box)

"White Castle. What you crave."

Source: http://www.ffood.net/fast_food_slogans.htm

OK We get it

Just one more point. Even the USDA, stumbled and failed. Sure, they put up a few "eat five" signs in grocery stores. But they also came out with The Food Guide Pyramid. A guide to Daily Food Choices, which is constantly featured in magazines and newspapers, and is used as a guide by dieticians. According to US. Government nutrition experts, the foundation of a healthy diet is "bread, cereal, rice and pasta." I am not making this up. This is a direct quote:

Use the Pyramid to help you eat better every day... the Dietary Guidelines way. Start with plenty of breads, cereals, rice and pasta...[4]

The Food Guide Pyramid suggests "Six to eleven servings" from this food group, and since they offer no advice on the types of bread, cereal, rice and pasta, Mr. Jones could start his day with a bowl of Choco Sugar-Frosted Bomb Flakes, have a bagel and coffee on his way to work, instant noodle lunch from the vending machine, and macaroni and (artificial) cheese for dinner.

Food Guide Pyramid

A Guide to Daily Food Choices

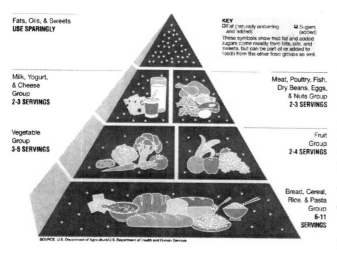

Fats, Oils, & Sweets
USE SPARINGLY

KEY
☐ Fat (naturally occurring and added)   ☐ Sugars (added)
These symbols show that fat and added sugars come mostly from fats, oils, and sweets, but can be part of or added to foods from the other food groups as well.

Milk, Yogurt, & Cheese Group
2-3 SERVINGS

Meat, Poultry, Fish, Dry Beans, Eggs, & Nuts Group
2-3 SERVINGS

Vegetable Group
3-5 SERVINGS

Fruit Group
2-4 SERVINGS

Bread, Cereal, Rice, & Pasta Group
6-11 SERVINGS

SOURCE: U.S. Department of Agriculture/U.S. Department of Health and Human Services

And according to the Food Guide Pyramid, he'd still need up to seven more servings of starch...so, maybe a few rolls with his lunch or half a box of crackers while watching TV.

I'm not a conspiracy nut, but you have to wonder what's going on. Where did this pyramid come from? Oh right. Experts from a handful of nutrition think tanks, the two most prominent being The American Society for Nutrition in Bethesda, Maryland, and the International Life Sciences Institute (ILSI) in Washington DC.

And while these are fine organizations that both publish important books and journals, they have a peculiar, rather unscientific financial base: corporate sponsorships.

Here are the "Sustaining Members" of the American Society for Nutrition:

The National Cattlemen's Beef Association (NCBA)

Coca-Cola Company

ConAgra Foods, Inc.

General Mills

Kellogg Company

Kraft Foods

Mars, Inc.

McDonald's

Monsanto

National Dairy Council

Nestle

PepsiCo

Pfizer

Procter & Gamble

Salt Institute

Sara Lee Corporation

The Sugar Association, Inc.

Tate & Lyle

Welch's

And here are the Corporate Sponsors of the International Life Sciences Institute, whose "activities focus primarily on nutrition and health promotion; food safety; risk assessment; and the environment."[5]

Coca Cola

PepsiCo

Mars, Incorporated

Kraft Foods

Dow Agro Sciences /The Dow Chemical Company

Monsanto

Kellogg

Red Bull

McDonalds

National Starch Foods

Procter & Gamble

Wrigley Confectionery

ExxonMobil Biomedical Sciences

Shell Chemicals, Ltd.

General Mills

Archer Daniels Midland

Cadbury Adams

ConAgra Foods

Dr Pepper Snapple Group

The Hershey Company

Corn Products International

Sara Lee Corporation

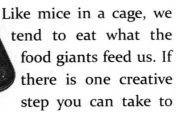

Like mice in a cage, we tend to eat what the food giants feed us. If there is one creative step you can take to improve your health, it is to leave the cage (it's not locked) and think for yourself.

On *The Metabolic Makeover*, reducing carbs is surprisingly easy. After all, most of the carbs we ingest are completely worthless anyway, so there is no worry about missing essential nutrients. In addition, most people on *The Metabolic Makeover* report a dramatic reduction in carb cravings, so there's no feeling of deprivation.

What's a reasonable amount of carbs?

That depends on your size and your activity level. For most active adults, keeping carbs below 100g per day will greatly help your Metabolic Makeover 70 to 80g per day is ideal for most people, and still allows for a wide range of whole grains, fruits and vegetables. In fact, with the exception of high-carb veggies like potatoes and yams, you can eat as many vegetables as you want. We are, after all, hunters and gatherers, remember?

What are Net Carbs?

Since fiber is included in the carbohydrate count on food labels, but is essentially non-digestible, the net-carb number is total carbs minus the fiber. Thus if you look at a can of beans, you might see the carbs per serving listed as 20g. But beans are also high in fiber, with a ½ cup serving providing about 9g! Thus the net-carb value of that food would be 11g, certainly a good food choice.

A slice of whole-grain bread will have a net-carb value of about 8g. Let's compare that to a jelly doughnut, with zero fiber and about 30g of carbs more than half of which is pure sugar.

Some people find that reducing carbs is as easy as avoiding anything made with flour. Other people use any of the carb counters available on the internet, or an app for your smart phone.

Bottom line, most people see dramatic improvements with carb intake less than 100g per day. As you reduce your carbohydrate intake, you are likely to experience:

- Less puffiness, especially around your eyes
- Fewer wrinkles
- Better digestion (less bloating, flatulence)
- Disapproval of carboholic friends

Now that you're "carb-conscious," let's move on to other dietary factors.

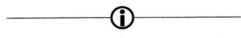

Summary

1. The three "whammies," insulin resistance, elevated glucose (blood sugar) and Inflammation, create a vicious cycle leading to Type 2 Diabetes, obesity, heart disease and cancer. In other words, the cause of death for 8 out of 10 people.

2. The body creates triglycerides (combination of glucose and fat) as a storage form of energy. This is great if you're active. If you're sedentary, high levels of triglycerides in the blood contributes directly to heart and blood vessel disease.

3. Another vicious cycle is created as adipose cells off-load fat into adjacent muscle. This damages the muscle so it is less able to use fat as fuel.

4. Most people achieve excellent results (maintaining ideal weight, high metabolic efficiency, energy and stamina) by keeping total carbs under 100g per day. Ideal is 70-80g per day.

5. Obviously, athletes and people who are very physically active can consume more than 100 grams of carbohydrate. In fact, many endurance athletes prepare for events by "carbo-loading" with 500 grams or more of starch, which they subsequently burn up in competition.

Endnotes

1   Yang YX, Hennessy S, Lewis JD. Insulin therapy and colorectal cancer risk among type 2 diabetes mellitus patients. Gastroenterology. 2004 Oct;127(4):1044-50.

2   Exp Diabetes Res. 2012;2012:789174. Epub 2012 Jun 4. Insulin resistance and cancer risk: an overview of the pathogenetic mechanisms. Arcidiacono B, Iiritano S, Nocera A, Possidente K, Nevolo MT, Ventura V, Foti D, Chiefari E, Brunetti A.

3   http://www.sciencedaily.com/releases/2011/07/110705123342.htm

4   http://www.nal.usda.gov/fnic/Fpyr/pmap.htm

5   http://www.ilsi.org/

Chapter Five

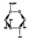

FOOD AS INFORMATION

The DNA era started for me in 2000, when we installed a full-scale genomics lab in our research facility. Suddenly, we were able to look beyond the nutrient content of a food, to observe the effect of plant compounds at the DNA level. In Chapter One I explained how the human genome is constantly adjusting to your diet, environment and situation. Genomics allowed us to understand and measure these changes.

For over three years, we searched through our medicinal plant library for compounds with clear metabolic benefits. With the aid of high-speed screening technologies like LCMS and GCMS, we discovered plant compounds that sent important metabolic instructions to the genome.

Everyone knows that drugs like amphetamines (and to a lesser extent, caffeine) can stimulate the nervous system and create the illusion of energy. But we were looking for non-stimulant effects that influence how the body creates, stores and uses energy. We focused on the most relevant metabolic "switches," or compounds, Adiponectin and AMPK.

Adiponectin: A protein secreted by fat cells, which tells the body to:

1. Burn more fat
2. Make less fat
3. Improve insulin sensitivity

AMPK: Considered to be the "master switch," AMPK is an enzyme secreted mainly in the liver and muscles that tells the body to:

1. Burn more fat
2. Make less fat
3. Make more glycogen
4. Increase energy production in muscle cells. Can you say mitochondrial biogenesis?

If you're wondering why these amazing compounds are not available at your drug or health-food store, it's because they are large, fragile proteins that would be digested long before they could reach your bloodstream. Nor can they be injected safely.

A number of pharmaceutical drugs have AMPK and Adiponectin-like activity. These include metformin, a drug used to treat type-2 diabetes, a group of drugs known as TZD's (thiazolidinediones) and an experimental drug known as AICAR.

If you would rather use natural products to optimize AMPK and Adiponectin, there are plenty, as described in Chapter Eight, Metabolic Modifiers.

Natalie note
It is often the case that synthetic drugs act like a sledgehammer in the human body. Drugs produce dramatic results, but often equally drastic side effects. The natural approach is more like a screwdriver, making adjustments to restore balance. In the case of energy

metabolism; whether the body burns glucose or stored fat, the natural approach has been remarkably safe and effective. Nutritional metabolic modifiers have been discovered that influence fat burning, exercise tolerance, strength, stamina, body composition and overall health. This is a core feature of *The Metabolic Makeover*.

Your Dinner is Talking to Your Cells

In the last decade, more than 12,000 studies were published documenting the effect of food and herbal compounds at the DNA level. The message is loud and clear. Food is information. What you eat alters your genes. And when I share these insights with people, it tends to make them think twice about the triple bacon cheeseburger, because the message that sends to your body is "EMERGENCY!" And if you're eating that nearly indigestible mass of hormone- and drug-laced saturated fat while you're driving, the alarm is twice as loud and the effect—in terms of the production of stress hormones like cortisol—is profound. If only people could hear the stress that is created by what and how they eat.

Can we all agree on a simple rule? No eating while driving. Studies show that simply getting behind the wheel of a car dramatically reduces digestive efficiency. And don't forget the dangers of taking your eyes off the road in order to keep the grease, ketchup and mayonnaise from dripping on your clothes.

So if food and behavior sends information to the genome, what is the best way to eat? Once again, the answer has to do with the diet and behavior that we are designed for.

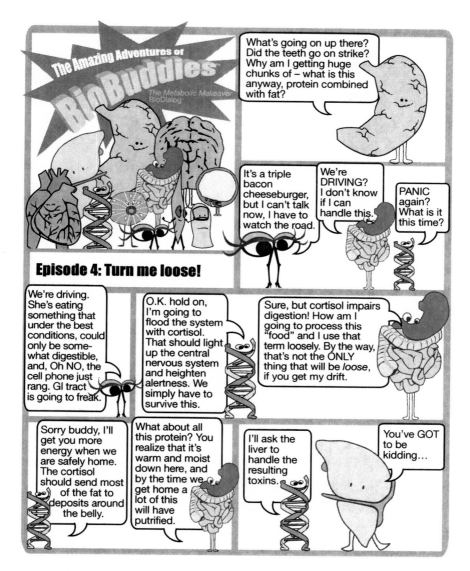

We're not saying you should go out in the woods and gather roots, berries, and tender shoots, but let's identify the characteristics of a hunting and gathering diet and match those with food choices that are readily available. There are three key points...

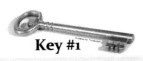

My research with hunter/gatherers cataloged 75 plant species in their daily diet. Imagine the astounding number of nutrients provided by such a diet! The average American consumes 11 species of plants in a week; meaning that hundreds of receptors, transport proteins and binding sites are deprived of their assigned compound. How about a metaphor to help illustrate this point?

When you land at an airport, you see nicely-dressed men and women holding signs with people's names on them. These limo drivers are waiting for a specific passenger. If that passenger doesn't show up, the limo driver leaves, and all of the business that was going to take place doesn't happen.

In your gastrointestinal tract and throughout your body, there are receptors and transport proteins holding "signs" for nutrients that never show up. And all of the biochemical "business" that these compounds were supposed to conduct does not happen.

We're not talking about vitamins for which there are clear deficiency diseases. But these plant compounds (called secondary metabolites) are still essential for peak health. Without them, your hair will not fall out. You won't get rickets or beriberi. But you won't look, feel or perform as well as you could.

We tend to eat what our mothers prepared. We eat what we like. We get into food ruts that last a lifetime, until our awareness changes. Take this simple step. Add one new vegetable to your shopping cart every month. Select from:

- Kale
- Chard
- Kohlrabi
- Celeriac (aka celery root)
- Beets
- Bok Choy

- Mustard greens
- Arugula
- Radicchio
- Turnips (root and greens)
- Asparagus
- Daikon
- Leeks
- Anise

- Cilantro
- Romanesco
- Eggplant
- Chayote squash
- Spaghetti squash
- Acorn squash
- Brussels sprouts
- Broccoli sprouts

NOTE: Alfalfa sprouts are not on this list for two reasons:

1. Negligible nutritional value
2. Frequent contamination with E. coli bacteria

Adding more vegetables into your diet has never been easier. Today, the produce section of most all supermarkets offer pre-washed and pre-cut vegetables, along with a variety of ready-made salads and leafy greens.

A few tips on getting your family to eat more vegetables.

1. You can poach vegetables

You can use water, but why not some chicken broth and white wine? Bring your liquid to a boil, add cut vegetables, and boil for only about 5 minutes. Your veggies will still be bright-ly-colored and crisp. Season as desired.

2. You can roast vegetables

In our home, if anything is going in the oven, like a chicken, it is never alone. Right next to it in a baking dish are cut vegetables. And the sky's the limit. Some of our favorites are zucchini, bell peppers, carrots, beets, sliced turnips, eggplant, asparagus, peeled garlic, thickly-sliced onion and, of course, broccoli. Drizzle olive oil and desired spices on the vegetables and roast at 375 ° for about 20 minutes. Don't overcook. Your veggies should not be mushy.

3. Make salads exciting

In restaurants, have you ever been surprised at the ingredients in your salad? It's like a taste adventure to see the standard variety of greens with added ingredients like walnuts, sliced pears, arugula, radicchio, green peas and cilantro.

4. Blender magic

You need a high-quality blender. You may not think you do, but once you own one, you'll wonder how you lived without it. Vitamix® and Ninja® are the most popular. Both use high-powered motors that can "blenderize" just about anything. That means soup in a matter of minutes, sauces, dips and green smoothies. Fruit smoothies require some protein because the natural sugars can get pretty high when you're using fruits like banana, mango and pineapple.

Our kids use the Vitamix every day, often experimenting with leftover veggies and a variety of spices. They also make healthy ice cream out of almonds, whey protein, and whatever fruit is in season. Late summer, the entire Pacific Northwest is busting with berries, cherries, apples and pears.

5. Healthy desserts

Fruit makes a great dessert, and our favorite topper will surprise and delight you. Open a can of organic, unsweetened coconut milk. You'll find that the fat has separated from the liquid. Scoop out some of the pure coconut fat and simply whip with a spoon or whisk. This topping is already sweet, but if you absolutely must sweeten it, use some Xylitol or Stevia.

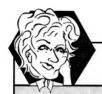

Why did hunter/gatherers eat so many plants?

Plants don't run away.
(Pa dum bum. I'm here all week.)

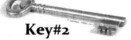 **Key#2   Eat Uncooked Foods as Often as Possible**

Between 2001 and 2011, more than 9,000 cookbooks were published in the United States. That's nine thousand more than were published in the first two million years of human existence. Cooking, in other words, although extremely popular, is a fairly new development, and one that destroys some vitamins—most notably, antioxidants—before they make it to our mouths.

That doesn't mean that you should never cook food. Cooking meat (the oldest form of cooking) is important for food safety. Not only did cooking meat destroy microbes, it made meat (and many plants) more digestible, which significantly increased the energy available to our calorie-starved ancestors.[1]

Cooking is also one of life's pleasures. However, it is wise to consume most of your plant foods in their raw natural state. Regarding complex meals where vegetables are combined with meat, poultry or fish, it is best to use a cooking style like stir-frying (i.e., with a wok) rather than exposing the food to high temperatures for long periods of time.

What about a raw diet?

Many people choose a raw-food diet. And while I certainly respect their decision, it bothers me that there is so much misinformation associated with that lifestyle. Perhaps the most pervasive myth is that cooking destroys valuable enzymes that are required for the optimal digestion of food.

Plants do contain enzymes, but none of these play an important role in human physiology. The simple truth is that plant enzymes do plant things and human enzymes do human things. If plant enzymes had biological activity in your body, eating a banana might cause brown spots to appear on your skin.

But dozens of books have been written about the importance of preserving the enzyme content of food.

That does not mean the material in those books, articles and websites is accurate. For decades, I have been asking raw-food enthusiasts to name one plant enzyme that I need to lead a long and extremely healthy life. I'm still waiting.

My recommendation for eating food as close as possible to its raw, natural state is to retain nutrients and prevent the formation of toxins that result from high-heat cooking. Particularly noteworthy are: Advanced Glycation End products (AGE's) and Acrylamide.

AGE's form when a sugar (primarily glucose and fructose) binds to a protein. This process—also called glycation or cross-linking—alters the protein. And since proteins are involved in thousands of biochemical activities throughout the body, glycation is now considered a major cause of the degeneration that accompanies "normal" aging.

I thought protein just made muscle.

That's a common belief, but listen to this: A major portion of every metabolic process in your body depends on the perfect timing of more than 50 thousand proteins. Enzymes are proteins that catalyze chemical reactions in every cell and tissue. Glycated enzymes don't work. Proteins turn genes off and on, carry nutrients and other essential biochemicals throughout the body, help balance blood chemistry, play an integral role in the immune system, and direct the entire process of cell repair. When these proteins are glycated, they become less soluble and tend to clump. In fact, glycated proteins appear to be a major component of the plaque that causes Alzheimer's disease.[2] Cataracts are another example, where cross-linked proteins in the lens of the eye cause vision loss.

Anti-Glycation Action Steps

1. Since AGE's are formed when a sugar binds a protein, it only makes sense to reduce your intake of all refined sugars. NOTE: Fructose glycates proteins faster than any other type of sugar.[3]

Diabetics age faster than non-diabetics because their elevated blood sugar accelerates the formation of AGE's, most notably an AGE known as Glycosylated Hemoglobin or HgbA1C.

2. Since heat accelerates the formation of AGE's, it only makes sense to limit high-heat cooking.

* Limit browned or charred foods. This includes grilled or barbecued meat, poultry and fish, as well as well-done broiled meats. Evidence is mounting that consumption of well-cooked (not even charred) meat is associated with increased risk for breast cancer.[4]

* Don't overcook eggs. This doesn't mean you should eat eggs raw or runny [that increases risk for salmonella] but avoid cooking them to death. Avoid the eternally re-heated scrambled eggs at breakfast buffets.

* Most foods contain some protein that can be glycated. Thus even burned toast contains some level of AGE material.

* Cook foods at the lowest possible temperature. Deep-frying is the worst not only because of the excessive heat but the incorporation of high amounts of fat. Oxidized fats increase the risk for deposits of lipofuscin, which leads to "age spots" on the skin and other tissues of the body. Thus poaching, microwaving, steaming, stir-frying and careful broiling (to avoid charring) are preferred.

The related toxin produced by heat is acrylamide.

In April 2002, a Swedish study was presented at a biomedical conference which created a stir among toxicologists around the world. Scientists testing a long list of starchy foods cooked with high heat found extremely high levels of acrylamide, a cancer-causing chemical.[5] They proposed that the toxin is formed whenever starches are exposed to high heat.

Weeks later, a British team confirmed the findings, looking at fried, baked and processed foods such as French fries, potato chips, corn chips, biscuits and "puffed" breakfast cereals. The results so alarmed health experts—they found acrylamide levels a thousand times higher than international safety limits—that a flurry of research soon followed.

A decade later, after scores of studies, there has been no glaring association found between acrylamide levels and any type of cancer. Food safety organizations are stating that "acrylamide in food is unlikely to pose a health risk."[6] But the word "unlikely" makes me think that it is prudent to reduce intake of processed carbohydrates, whether baked, puffed or fried. Most of these fall into the category of "junk food" anyway, because they are high in fat (often the worst kind of fat), high in sodium, and provide no significant vitamins, minerals, or fiber.

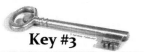

Key #3   Eat Smaller, More-Frequent Meals

Hunter/gatherers ate when they were hungry and stopped eating when their hunger was satisfied. This meant roughly 250 to 300 calories for an active tribesperson per meal; the amount we civilized folks normally consume before the entree. In reality, it takes a small quantity of food to satisfy hunger. If you don't believe this, try it yourself. Next time you're hungry, eat slowly and chew well. Notice that the subtle aromas of the food intensify the longer you chew. Be sensitive to the point when your hunger is gone. Most people find it's somewhere between one third to one half of the meal.

There are two reasons for our tendency to eat beyond hunger satisfaction, the first being that we eat too fast. It takes about 20 minutes for your brain to get the message (via the hormone

Cholecystokinin) that hunger has been satisfied. So, when you eat quickly, it is very easy to overeat. You may even feel hungry the entire time you're eating, so you consume more than you need. Eating in a slow and relaxed manner gives your brain time to receive the message that you've consumed an adequate amount of food.

Slow Down! The pre-meal stomach is quite acidic, and the ingestion of food dilutes or buffers that acid. Effective digestion depends upon the stomach's ability to re-acidify during a meal, and the slower you eat, the better. Adequate stomach acid activates gastric enzymes and initiates protein breakdown. Try this: after every bite, put down your spoon or fork and chew thoroughly. Don't pick up your utensil, until your mouth is completely empty. Take sips of water between bites.

We also tend to overeat because we know our next meal is four to five hours away. Hunter/gatherers don't operate on this schedule. They will eat again in an hour or two if they get hungry. The hunter/gatherer style of eating, which could be called grazing, is the most efficient way to eat. Studies show that people who consume 2,000 calories per day via grazing tend to lose weight, while people eating the same number of calories at lunch and dinner (as 90% of Americans do) tend to gain weight. Digestion, nutrient absorption, and metabolism all tend to improve with smaller, more frequent meals.

The grazing vs. gorging issue was examined by Dr. Emanuel Cheraskin in an excellent review of the scientific literature. Grazing tends to improve blood lipids (mainly triglycerides) as well as glucose and insulin balance.[7] Importantly, these short-term improvements can certainly be expected to contribute to long-term benefits, including reduced risk for obesity, diabetes and heart disease.

You can get in the habit of grazing by keeping healthful snacks in the office or around the house. Fresh vegetables and fruit are good choices. I use a powdered "green drink" mixed in a glass of water mid-morning and mid-afternoon. My favorite contains a long list of organic, dehydrated high-nutrient vegetables including: wheat grass, barley grass, cruciferous vegetables, tomato powder, garlic and spirulina. This not only satisfies my hunger, but provides the phytonutrient equivalent of four or five bowls of salad.

Using this snacking or "grazing" strategy allows you to arrive home in the evening without the ravenous hunger that causes so much overeating at night. You'll find it easy to consume smaller portions because your body's energy needs have been satisfied consistently throughout the day. Your blood sugar levels will be stabilized, and as a result, your energy level and mood will remain steady rather than swinging wildly up and down.

The manner in which we ingest calories (fuel) clearly sends important messages to the genome regarding how to handle the caloric load. Grazing is far more likely to send a "convert fuel to energy" message. Large meals on the other hand, exceed the energy needs of the body, resulting in a biological imperative to convert calories to fat.

More Signals: The Protein/Carb Ratio

As we've explained, the hunting/gathering diet was nearly devoid of pure carbohydrate. Aside from the rare discovery of a beehive, virtually all carbs were accompanied by significant amounts of fat, protein, and fiber. That mix works quite well even today, since the signals from these macronutrients tend to balance each other out.

Carbs stimulate the secretion of insulin, which tells the body to store calories. Protein has a modest effect on insulin, but mainly stimulates glucagon, a hormone that directs the liver to release energy. Fat tends to slow down both processes, and fiber improves nearly every phase of digestion and elimination.

The avalanche of concentrated and refined, low-fiber carbohydrate in the modern Western diet creates an enormous challenge for you and me. To remain healthy, and to have a prayer of maintaining ideal weight, we have to make a few critical adjustments to the mix of foods in every meal.

In her note in Chapter Three, Natalie advised, "Never eat unopposed carbs." She pointed out that protein, fat and fiber reduce the glycemic response—the rate at which a food raises blood sugar. New research reveals another glucose-lowering advantage for protein. We now know that protein (especially the branched chain amino acids) signals the muscles to take up glucose and convert it to that wonderful energy reserve compound known as glycogen.[8,9]

Protein also has a profound effect on appetite. Dr. Alison Gosby and a group of researchers at the University of Sydney's School of Biological Sciences found that consuming adequate protein, rather than simply cutting calories, is the key to prevent overeating. They explain that animals have separate appetites for carbohydrates, fat and protein; and that "If protein in the diet is diluted, even by a small amount by extra carbohydrate, the appetite for protein dominates and [animals] will keep eating in an attempt to attain their target level of protein."[10]

> *"Our findings have considerable implications for body weight management in the current nutritional environment, where foods rich in fat and carbohydrates are cheap, often addictive, and available to an extent unprecedented in human history."*
>
> ~ Dr. Alison Gosby, School of Biological Sciences, University of Sydney, Australia

Bottom line: The title of this chapter refers to food as information. But remember that it is not just the composition of the food that affects your genome, but the quantity of food, the balance of carbohydrate and protein, and the way that it is consumed. Obviously, some foods are more valuable than others. Here's our list of Superfoods that have important conversations with your genome.

Superfoods

1. The Allium family of vegetables

Alliums include garlic, garlic shoots, onions, leeks, shallots, chives, and scallions. There isn't another group of plants that has more extensive and impressive scientific support for remarkable health benefits. Include small amounts of alliums in your daily diet instead of loading up once or twice a week. Evidence gathered in the Iowa Women's Health Study suggests that one third to one half of a clove of garlic per day was sufficient to confer a whopping 50% reduction in risk to colon cancer.[11]

Intake of alliums has been associated with decreased risk for cancer of the skin, stomach, liver, lungs, and cervix. Research suggests that the major signaling molecules include more than

70 different sulfur compounds which tell the body to create the powerful immune and detox protein known as glutathione. Red onions also contain quercetin, a flavonoid with antioxidant and anticancer activity.

2. The cabbage-broccoli family (Brassica)

Cabbage, Brussels sprouts, kale, turnips, turnip greens, collard greens, broccoli, cauliflower, rutabaga, kohlrabi, and radishes all contain powerful compounds known as indoles and Isothiocyanates, which boost immune protection against illness. Researchers have even identified how these food compounds talk to your DNA to reduce your risk for cancer.[12]

3. Carrots, sweet potatoes, and yams

Nature has a wonderful way of pointing to extraordinarily valuable foods. Deep orange, yellow and red colors indicate the presence of carotenoids, compounds that are associated with significant health benefits. Carotenoids with names like beta-carotene, beta-cryptoxanthin, lutein and zeaxanthin are powerful antioxidants. Alpha carotene, beta carotene, and beta cryptoxanthin can be converted by the body into Vitamin A.

Your grandmother knew that carrots were good for the eyes. We now know why. The lens and retina of your eyes actually contain lutein and zeaxanthin, and research suggests that consumption of carotenoid-rich foods may help prevent age-related macular degeneration and cataracts.[13] Carrots, sweet potatoes and yams also provide healthy amounts of beta carotene, vitamin C, calcium, magnesium, and fiber.

NOTE: Get your carotenoids from food sources. In 3 intervention studies, beta-carotene supplements were associated with increases in lung cancer, cardiovascular diseases, and total mortality among smokers. Thus, Natalie and I do not recommend beta-carotene supplements for anyone who has ever smoked cigarettes.[14]

4. Tomatoes and tomato products

Tomatoes contain a carotenoid known as lycopene, and studies have revealed an apparent anti-cancer benefit. Scientists looking for an association between specific foods and disease risk (epidemiologists) report that lycopene-rich diets are associated with significant reductions in the risk of prostate cancer.[15] And it looks like tomato products are the most valuable source of lycopene. In a study looking at the diet history of 47,000 male health professionals, those with the highest intakes of tomatoes and tomato products had a risk of prostate cancer that was 35% lower and a risk of aggressive prostate cancer that was a whopping 53% lower than those with the lowest lycopene consumption. [16]

Why not just take lycopene supplements?

Because there are very likely other compounds in tomato that contribute to these benefits. There is no known danger associated with lycopene supplements, but it only makes sense to take advantage of what we know. Tomato is a bona fide superfood.

5. Berries and Cherries

The deep blue and purple color indicates the presence of a group of powerful antioxidants known as anthocyanins. The anthocyanin pigments of Bilberries (Vaccinium myrtillus) have long been used for improving vision and circulation. There is also evidence that certain anthocyanins have anti-inflammatory properties, and there are reports that anthocyanin-rich foods are beneficial for treating diabetes and ulcers.[17]

If that's not enough reason to consume berries, recent research has identified significant anti-bacterial and anti-viral activity, as well as the ability (in old animals) to restore balance, co-ordination, learning and memory.[18] Overall, a cup of blueberries per day can provide significant antioxidant and flavonoid benefits that may improve memory, mood, and cognition. Sugar-free berry concentrate drinks are also available which provide convenient high-potency nutrition for daily use.

6. Nuts and seeds

"Perhaps one of the most unexpected and novel findings in nutritional research in the past 5 years has been that nut consumption seems to protect against heart disease." So begins an excellent report in the *American Journal of Clinical Nutrition* showing that eating nuts reduces risk not only for heart disease but for all natural causes of death.[19] Seeds—especially sunflower, chia and flax seeds—may provide even greater benefit owing to their rich supply of antioxidant phenolic acids, artery-friendly essential fats, vitamin E, selenium, and anti-cancer lingans.

A SPECIAL NOTE ON ALMONDS:

- They're convenient
- A handful of almonds = 100 calories and will reduce appetite so much that you'll eat smaller meals, resulting in a net reduction of calories. Try having a handful of almonds 15 or 20 minutes before a meal.
- Helps stabilize blood sugar. Diabetics should never be more than an arms distance from a bag of almonds.
- Helps lower cholesterol
- A nutritional powerhouse!

- Contains essential fats
- Great source of magnesium (most Americans are deficient)
- 5g of protein in one handful of almonds
- Almond skins are loaded with antioxidant flavonoids.
- All forms of vitamin E (tocopherols)
- Good source of vitamin B2 (riboflavin)

Tip to get the MOST out of your almond experience:
- Buy ORGANIC unflavored almonds
- Soak overnight
- Drain water and place soaked almonds in a food dehydrator for 5-8 hours or until crunchy. Better than roasting. Easier to digest.
- Don't have a dehydrator? Place the soaked almonds on a cookie sheet and bake at 200° F for 2 hours.

7. Medicinal mushrooms

Fresh Shiitake mushrooms are available at most grocery stores and are also available dried in packages. Shiitakes contain a powerful immune-stimulating polysaccharide known as lentinan. Other power-packed medicinal mushrooms include: maitake, coriolus, and reishi, but even white button (agaricus) and portabella mushrooms provide significant health benefits.

8. Comprehensive "Green Drinks"

Powdered green drinks are readily available these days which can dramatically improve nutrition by providing hundreds of nutrients in a single serving. What's more, advanced processing technology can remove the non-nutritive cellulose, resulting in high-nutrient concentrates. Look for products that combine a variety of earth and sea vegetables and make sure all ingredients are organically grown.

Since green drinks tend to have a strong taste, manufacturers often "cut" the product with sweeteners and fillers. You want concentrated greens, not dextrose, maltodextrin or lecithin. Read labels carefully.

9. Cold-water fish

Mackerel, herring, smelt, anchovies, Icelandic cod, salmon, and sardines all provide valuable Omega-3 fatty acids (EPA & DHA), which can help prevent the formation of abnormal blood clots and decrease risk for heart disease. If you don't care for fish, 1,000mg of fish oil in capsules will approximate the benefits of a 3-ounce serving of fish.

NOTE: Consult with your physician if you are taking a blood-thinning medication such as warfarin, as the natural blood-thinning activity of fish oil may have an additive effect.

10. Olive oil

Reduce your use of butter (which is high in saturated fat) and throw out the highly-processed margarine made with hydrogenated oils. Forget the polyunsaturated corn and safflower oils. Instead, enjoy the rich and mellow flavor of first-press, virgin olive oil. Olive oil provides vitamin E and heart-healthy monounsaturated fats, and can help lower cholesterol.

11. Green peas

There's a wonder food just waiting for you in the freezer section of your grocery store: frozen peas. Frozen green peas are picked and packaged so fast that they have virtually the same nutritional value as fresh peas. A three-quarter cup serving contains 6 grams of protein, less than 1 gram of fat, 3.5 grams of fiber, and 35 mg of calcium. They're packed with folic acid, and antioxidants such as vitamin C and lutein. Lunch box tip:

if you pack a salad, top it off with frozen peas. They will thaw by lunchtime and keep your salad fresh and cold in the meantime.

12. Bran cereals

You've heard these cereals recommended for their fiber content, but that's not the half of it. Bran cereals like All-Bran®, Bran Buds® and 100% Bran® also contain high amounts of phytic acid or IP-6 This compound has been shown to support the immune system and significantly reduce risk for heart disease and cancer.[20]

13. Spices

Your spice rack probably contains at least five items that have powerful disease-preventing activity. Some, like cumin and turmeric act by reducing inflammation. Others like rosemary and oregano, are powerful antioxidants with remarkable anti-microbial activity. Garlic is in a class by itself, with known benefits for immunity, cardiovascular health and cancer prevention.

Another immune stimulant, chili peppers (cayenne, capsicum) can help ward off a cold and may reduce your risk for other, more serious illnesses. Cayenne has been shown to help prevent cardiovascular disease and the high flavonoid content may help prevent certain forms of cancer. Suggested use: be careful! Some types of chili peppers are extremely hot. Sprinkle in soup; salad dressing; Italian, Mexican, or Asian cuisine. For a morning pick-me-up, mix 1/4 tsp. in eggs or orange juice.

14. Dark green leafy vegetables

The only leafy vegetable many people eat is lettuce, a nutritional light-weight. Try to include kale, chard, spinach, arugula, beet tops and mustard greens in your diet. These longevity foods are packed with minerals, vitamins, carotenoids, flavonoids and perhaps most importantly, folic acid.

15. Avocados

The avocado (botanically, a berry with a single seed) is a true superfood. Loaded with healthy fats, potassium, fiber, and a raft of vitamins, this versatile food is even a good source of protein. Research at the UCLA Center for Human Nutrition has documented the ability of avocado to lower cholesterol, fight diabetes and reduce cancer risk.[21]

16. Industrial hemp

When I talk about the astounding nutritional value of hemp, most of my colleagues think this is something new. In fact, hemp is the oldest superfood on this list, with cultivation records going back thousands of years.

Hemp seeds contain high-quality protein, and while some food scientists complain about the yield (hemp seed is "only" 50% protein, compared to whey, where the protein content can exceed 90%), I hasten to point out that the other 50% of the seed is just as valuable.

Hemp is an excellent source of essential fats, vitamins, minerals, dietary fiber, and a raft of compounds that support immunity, gastrointestinal, and cardiovascular health.

See if whey (or any other protein source) can match this:

- Essential fatty acids, with the perfect Omega 3/6/9 ratio for human health
- Complete protein, providing all 22 amino acids
- Dietary fiber with the perfect insoluble/soluble ratio for GI health and cholesterol management

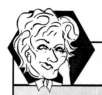

Why are hemp products (hemp "hearts," hemp protein, and hemp oil) so expensive?

Because all of it has to be imported. It is currently illegal to grow industrial hemp in the United States, even though Canadian farmers have been growing it since 1998 and now have more than 39,000 acres devoted to this superfood.

As we vote with our dollars and support hemp farmers and processors, we are moving closer to the day when these products will be a staple component of a highly varied natural foods diet.

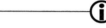

Summary

1. Keys to optimal health can be gained from research on hunters and gatherers:
   - Eat a wide variety of foods
   - Eat uncooked, or barely cooked foods as often as possible
   - Eat smaller, more frequent meals (grazing)

2. We all have limitations on the amount of food we can digest and metabolize. So it only makes sense to focus on what is most valuable, by reducing or eliminating junk calories and incorporating as many superfoods as possible into your diet.

3. High-heat cooking produces toxins related to accelerated aging, vision loss, Alzheimer's Disease, and cancer. Limit char-broiling and eliminate deep frying.

Endnotes

1 See: Catching Fire: How Cooking Made Us Human, by Richard Wrangham, Director of biological anthropology at Harvard University.

2 Smith MA, Taneda S, Richey PL, Miyata S, Yan SD, Stern D, Sayre LM, Monnier VM, Perry G. Advanced Maillard reaction end products are associated with Alzheimer disease pathology. Proc Natl Acad Sci U S A. 1994 Jun 7;91(12):5710-4.

3 Dills WL. Protein fructosylation: Fructose and the Maillard reaction. Am J Clin Nutr 1993; 58(suppl):779S-787S.

4 Zheng W, Gustafson DR, Sinha R, Cerhan JR, Moore D, Hong CP, Anderson KE, Kushi LH, Sellers TA, Folsom AR. Well-done meat intake and the risk of breast cancer. J Natl Cancer Inst. 1998 Nov 18;90(22):1724-9.

5 Acrylamide in food. Wkly Epidemiol Rec. 2002 May 17;77(20):166-

6 http://www.foodsafetynews.com/2012/01/panel-acrylamide-in-food-un-likely-to-pose-health-risk/

7 The Breakfast/ Lunch/ Dinner Ritual:
   http://orthomolecular.org/library/jom/1993/pdf/1993-v08n01-p006.pdf

8 Bernard JR, Liao YH, Hara D, Ding Z, Chen CY, Nelson JL, Ivy JL. An amino acid mixture improves glucose tolerance and insulin signaling in Sprague-Dawley rats. Am J Physiol Endocrinol Metab. 2011 Apr;300(4):E752-60.

9 Wang B, Kammer LM, Ding Z, Lassiter DG, Hwang J, Nelson JL, Ivy JL. Amino acid mixture acutely improves the glucose tolerance of healthy overweight adults. Nutr Res. 2012 Jan;32(1):30-8.

10 Gosby AK, Conigrave AD, Lau NS, Iglesias MA, Hall RM, et al. (2011) Testing Protein Leverage in Lean Humans: A Randomised Controlled Experimental Study. PLoS ONE 6(10): e25929. doi:10.1371/journal.pone.0025929

11 Steinmetz KA, et al. Vegetables, fruit and colon cancer in the Iowa Women's Health Study. Am J Epidemiol. 1994; 139;1, pg1-15

12 Gerhauser C. Epigenetic impact of dietary isothiocyanates in cancer chemoprevention. Curr Opin Clin Nutr Metab Care. 2013 Jul;16(4):405-10.

13 Mares-Perlman JA, Millen AE, Ficek TL, Hankinson SE. The body of evidence to support a protective role for lutein and zeaxanthin in delaying chronic disease. Overview. J Nutr. 2002;132(3):518S-524S.

14   Virtamo J, Pietinen P, Huttunen JK, Korhonen P, Malila N, Virtanen MJ, Albanes D, Taylor PR, Albert P; ATBC Study Group. Incidence of cancer and mortality following alpha-tocopherol and beta-carotene supplementation: a postintervention follow-up. JAMA. 2003 Jul 23;290(4):476-85.

15   Giovannucci E. A review of epidemiologic studies of tomatoes, lycopene, and prostate cancer. Exp Biol Med (Maywood). 2002;227(10):852-859

16   Giovannucci E, Ascherio A, Rimm EB, Stampfer MJ, Colditz GA, Willett WC. Intake of carotenoids and retinol in relation to risk of prostate cancer. J Natl Cancer Inst. 1995;87(23):1767-1776.

17   Seeram, Navindra P. (2008). "Berry Fruits: Compositional Elements, Biochemical Activities, and the Impact of Their Intake on Human Health, Performance, and Disease". Journal of Agricultural and Food Chemistry 56 (3): 627–9.

18   Shukitt-Hale B, Galli RL, Meterko V, Carey A, Bielinski DF, McGhie T, Joseph JA. Dietary supplementation with fruit polyphenolics ameliorates age-related deficits in behavior and neuronal markers of inflammation and oxidative stress. Age (Dordr). 2005 Mar;27(1):49-57. doi: 10.1007/s11357-005-4004-9.

19   Sabate J, Haddad E, Tanzman JS, Jambazian P, Rajaram S. Serum lipid response to the graduated enrichment of a Step I diet with almonds: a randomized feeding trial. Am J Clin Nutr. 2003;77(6):1379-1384.

20   Henderson AJ, Ollila CA, Kumar A, Borresen EC, Raina K, Agarwal R, Ryan EP. Chemopreventive properties of dietary rice bran: current status and future prospects. Adv Nutr. 2012 Sep 1;3(5):643-53.

21   Qing-Yi Lu, Yanjun Zhang, Yue Wang, David Wang, Ru-po Lee, Kun Gao, Russell Byrns, and David Heber. California Hass Avocado: Profiling of Carotenoids, tocopherol, fatty acid, and fat content during maturation and from different growing areas. UCLA Center for Human Nutrition, Department of Medicine, David Geffen School of Medicine, University of California, Los Angeles, California

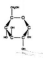

REFLECTIONS

NOW THAT YOU UNDERSTAND THE "INNER PART OF DINNER"...

1. Can you list three changes you'd like to make in your eating habits?

2. Any additions to your shopping list?

Notes:

Chapter Six

FOOD FADS AND FACTS

I've been studying the food/health relationship for 45 years, including a decade of clinical practice, nine years as a university instructor and 25 years of research. And I'm still learning, the reason being that the field is incredibly complex.

At the same time, we have amassed an enormous body of knowledge, and our understanding of the processes of digestion and metabolism is light years ahead of where it was just a few years ago. That's because we have new tools. We can peer inside the human body to analyze the effect of specific foods on the digestive tract and the immune system. Genomic analysis reveals specific gene variants that predispose some people to food-related problems like celiac disease. And we can measure specific molecules in the bloodstream that result in food allergy.

Importantly, I am part of an international scientific community where this information is continually discussed and refined through the process of peer review, conferences, webinars and thousands of websites—most of them interactive.

Not too many years ago, the submission of an important paper took 9 to 12 months to get to my desk due to weeks of peer review, editing the final manuscript, printing in a journal, mailing the journal to a few thousand subscribers, with the remainder sent to libraries (remember those?). Believe it or not, students and scientists could then check out the journal so that when others went looking, they would find every volume except the one they wanted.

Now, most journals publish electronically ahead of the print version, so the time it takes for important information to get to my computer screen has been reduced to a matter of days. What's more, automated retrieval services scan tens of thousands of papers every week and deliver any study to my inbox, published anywhere in the world, that relates to my particular area of interest.

Which means that an incredible amount of teamwork is required to manage and evaluate what is now a continual stream of new information. I am fortunate to work with such a team, including my wife, 22 scientists in the U.S. and 30 brilliant individuals in our lab in South Korea. I also manage a brain trust of health care professionals throughout North America who contribute clinical information to this effort, and that is distilled into our books and the website **www.TheMetabolicMakeover.com.**

So while it is easy to see how the Internet has accelerated the sharing of scientific knowledge, it is also true that the Internet has accelerated the sharing of misinformation, fad and folly. Many are calling this the "information age." I call it the confusion age, where anyone can say anything, and through the power of duplication – where material is forwarded at lightning speed to thousands of Internet users, it takes on the appearance of truth... even if it is utter nonsense.

I've written extensively on the importance of scientific integrity in this day and age; how people who write about health have a responsibility to follow guidelines that assure accuracy. But every bit of nonsense that is forwarded around the Internet is like a drop of poison in the well. If we—as a world community—are not careful, the entire well could be rendered undrinkable. "Webaloney," in other words, can reach the level where the average non scientist cannot discern truth from folly.

Every day I encounter people burdened by strong beliefs in things that are simply not true; things that have been debunked and actually proven false. When I politely ask where they got the "unusual" information, the invariable response is, "the Internet."

The Top 7 Food Controversies

Here are seven important topics that Natalie and I have thoroughly investigated:

1. SOY STORY

In the 80s and 90s, soy was the savior of mankind. It was going to replace meat, prevent cancer and heart disease, and feed a growing world population. Then in 2000, suddenly soy was poison. I was shocked at how far and how rapidly the pendulum swung; to the point where even educated people were scanning the ingredient list of everything they consumed in order to avoid eating a milligram of soy.

I don't mind the pendulum swinging a little. That's called self-correction. Common sense tells you that human beings are designed to eat a wide variety of protein sources. Making soy your major protein source could very well cause or contribute to significant health issues.

But the exaggeration and the intentional misrepresentation of research regarding soy was staggering. I'm happy to say that the pendulum is finally heading back to center. Here's what we believe that looks like:

Asians who eat a lot of soy have a lower incidence of certain cancers, most notably breast cancer and prostate cancer. But is there a causative relationship between consuming soybeans and a lower incidence of cancer or is it merely an association? In other words, I sing in the shower every morning and the sun rises. Does my singing cause the sun to rise, or do these events simply coincide? You get the picture.

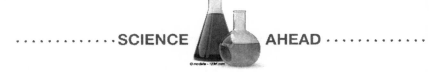

············SCIENCE AHEAD············

Scientists looking for causation found two components of soybeans with anti-cancer activity. The first are phytoestrogens, a group of compounds (e.g., genistein and daidzein) that have estrogen-like activity in humans and animals. Sometimes these are called isoflavones.

Soy phytoestrogens have very weak activity in humans. But because they bind to estrogen receptors in a woman's breasts and reproductive organs, it is believed that they block the binding of more powerful estrogens that she may be producing or getting from the environment. Strong estrogens can promote cancer. So there is a good chance that the lower cancer rates in Asian women relate to the blocking effect of phytoestrogens. In men, a similar benefit from soy may be achieved in the reduction of prostate cancer where estrogen plays a contributing role.

Second, scientists found a group of protease inhibitors in soy and other beans. These biochemicals inhibit the digestion of protein by interfering with the activity of two important enzymes, trypsin and chymotrypsin. Protease inhibitors interfere with cell communication, protein metabolism, and cell growth.[1] This may contribute to anti-cancer defense in humans by interfering with the growth and spread (metastasis) of tumors.

So we now have a reasonable cause and effect hypothesis between two biochemicals (phytoestrogens and protease inhibitors) and reduced cancer. What do we do with this valuable information?

Option one: We promote soy as the perfect food for all human beings, including infants.

Option two: We carefully evaluate the effects of phytoestrogens on pregnancy and fetal health. We evaluate the effects of phytoestrogens and protease inhibitors on the growth of children, and we look for possible side effects resulting from decreased estrogen binding. Estrogen, for example, plays an important role in the maintenance and repair of the brain.

For decades, many Americans pursued option one with wild abandon. Fueled by the burgeoning soybean industry and supported by thousands of health-food enthusiasts (motto: where's the next panacea?), the soy frenzy extended to the mass marketing of soy milk, soy protein, soy cheese, soy burgers, soy candy bars, soy butter (to replace peanut butter) and soy-enriched cereal, bread, pasta, and chips. Concentrates of soy phytoestrogens appeared in health food stores, and the FDA approved the health claim that 25 grams of soy protein per day could reduce risk for heart disease.

Then, new research (**self-correcting power of science**) started showing up.

The Metabolic Times

Vol. MCMXX, No. 144672

— FOUNDED 1881 —

Excessive Soy Consumption May Inhibit Brain Repair Functions

The basis for this concern arose when researchers documented a dampening effect of phytoestrogens on brain repair in rats.[2,3] Human studies appear to support this finding. A study with Japanese-Americans found a disturbing correlation between soy consumption and cognitive impairment.[4,5] I am not suggesting that soy = brain degeneration, but the issue certainly needs further study.

What doesn't need further study is the association between high soy consumption and growth and development. Here, the concern is that soy phytoestrogens may cause early puberty in girls and delayed physical maturation in boys. It was determined that the amount of phytoestrogens in a day's worth of soy infant formula had the same estrogenic effect as five birth-control pills to an adult.[6] A study published in the British medical journal *Lancet* found that infants who were fed soy formula had levels of phytoestrogens that were 13,000 to 22,000 times higher than natural estrogen concentrations in early life.[7]

Protease Inhibitors Found in Soy
May Inhibit Normal Growth

There is also concern that protease inhibitors found in soy foods may inhibit normal growth and repair functions in children. At first, the soy industry claimed that these inhibitors were destroyed by cooking, but many researchers disagreed. Protease inhibitors have been shown to survive cooking and processing to a small degree, but certainly significant enough for a growing child.[8]

Soy Linked to Thyroid

The thyroid factor may also create problems for children and adults who consume high amounts of soy foods. The phytoestrogens genistein and daidzein have been found to interfere with thyroid function,[9] and although this has been shown to have no effect on a person eating a varied diet, those using soy as their primary source of protein may suffer.[10]

The Isoflavone/Phytoestrogen Controversy

As we write this book, there is no scientific consensus regarding the effect of soy isoflavones on breast-cancer risk, or the benefits for women's health in general.

When Natalie and I examine the data from conflicting studies—well-conducted scientific investigations that arrive at opposite conclusions—we find a number of what are called confounding variables.

- There is no benchmark population to compare to the Western diet. Intake of isoflavones in North America is estimated to be between 0.5 and 3 mg per day.[11] Also, there is no "Asian diet." Even in the same country (Japan), you find people in the interior eating a lot more soy than people living on the coast, (who eat more fish) and people in the cities (who eat more meat). Thus daily isoflavone intake varies from 5 to more than 100 mg per day.

- Different soy foods provide different isoflavones. In fermented soy products like natto or tempeh, aglycones are the principal form of isoflavone, whereas in unfermented soy products, like tofu, soy milk or soy supplements, isoflavones are primarily present as glucosides. These different forms are absorbed and metabolized differently.

- At what age did soy food consumption begin, and/or how long should supplements be consumed? There is evidence that the reduction of breast cancer among Asian women is derived from the consumption of soy foods early in life. Likewise, the observed reduction in breast cancer in women consuming isoflavone supplements occurs mainly in postmenopausal women taking the supplements for more than 5 years.[12]

The Bottom Line on Soy

It's natural to jump on bandwagons. Nutrition is extremely complex and we would all love a simple solution to the threats of heart disease and cancer. But I'd like to suggest that in regard to soy foods, as in all things, moderation is the key.

- If you eat a lot of meat, you can do yourself and the planet a favor by switching to vegetable proteins at least a few days a week. That's not just soy foods, but any combination of beans, whole grains, organic dairy foods, nuts and seeds.

- If you are pregnant or nursing, soy should not be your major source of protein. Three to five servings per week appears to be safe, but please consult with your OB/GYN, midwife or pediatrician.

- Natalie and I advise against using soy formula for babies. If you absolutely cannot breastfeed, consult a qualified health professional to work out a rotation strategy using goat's milk, almond, rice and coconut milk.

- If you have growing children, make sure they have a variety of proteins in their diet. Soy is fine, but if it is their major protein, you may be limiting their adult height.

2. A GRAIN OF TRUTH

In Chapter Two, I presented a brief history of grain; how plants evolved to produce starchy seeds, and ultimately how that remarkably successful survival skill spread around the world by the wind and by the humans who discovered this powerful nutrient source. That occurred about 12,000 years ago, and grain soon became the "staff of life" because it could be stored and ground up to make portable foods like hardtack, flatbread and corncakes. It could be carried in sacks, mixed with water and heated to make gruel. From that point on, humans and plants co-evolved, and the list of grains expanded from a few to a few dozen.

BIG QUESTION: Are we really adapted to the grain-based diet that most people eat today? The evolutionary forces that produced our metabolic machinery were developed over millions of years. With that perspective, 12,000 years is the blink of an eye, and a growing number of scientists are questioning the wisdom of a grain-based diet.

Of course, you may say that the modern Western diet is not really "grain-based." We eat a wide variety of foods that include grains. But take a good look around at what people are eating.

* Millions of North American kids start their day with an onslaught of refined grains (breakfast cereal) containing more sugar than a candy bar.

* Millions of adults start their day with coffee and grains, either in the form of a doughnut, bagel (not much difference), croissant, muffin, scone, or bear claw.

* Lunch features grain in the form of a sandwich or hamburger bun, as well as the bag of corn chips.

* Dinner might be pasta or rice, more bread or another grain.

* Eating out? Every restaurant meal starts with bread and ends with a grain-based dessert.

* The vast majority of snack foods are made from corn or wheat.

Remember the USDA's Food Guide Pyramid from Chapter Four? The guide that recommended 6 to 11 servings from the "bread, cereal, rice and pasta" group? Guess what, in 2010, the average American consumed even more than that! According to USDA data, the average sedentary American now consumes more grain than is recommended for "teen-age boys or men who engage in heavy physical activity."[13]

That can't be good.

Important Definitions

Sugar is defined as any of several simple carbohydrates, divided primarily into monosaccharides (a single sugar unit, such as glucose or fructose), disaccharides (two sugar units, e.g., sucrose, a.k.a. table sugar) and polysaccharides (of which there are thousands) made up of repeating glucose units.

The term starch refers to polysaccharides consisting of a large number of glucose units joined together by strong beta linkages or weak alpha bonds.

To review: Your body can generate energy from carbohydrate, fat or protein. The easiest fuel is carbohydrate, supplied in chains of sugar units called saccharides. The smallest are monosaccharides such as blood sugar or glucose. Saccharide chains can also be massive, some linking hundreds of sugars. These are called polysaccharides. In the process of digestion, these enormous chains are broken down to smaller and smaller units that are absorbed and transported to the tissues of the body. The speed by which this occurs determines whether a carbohydrate produces a biochemical celebration (**"Yay, energy!"**) or alarm (**OVERLOAD, stress, pancreatic panic**).

It is not just the size or length of the polysaccharide chain that determines the speed by which glucose enters the bloodstream. The links that hold the chain together can be strong or weak, and the structure of the food itself can facilitate or slow down digestion.

The hunting/gathering diet provided carbohydrates from roots and tubers where the saccharides were in strong beta links and locked up in cellulose compartments. Thus there was a significant amount of work, both mechanical (chewing) and biochemical (digestion) that had to be done before those energy molecules could enter the bloodstream.

But grain is very different. The saccharides in grain are held together by alpha-linkages, which are easily broken, and soon after discovering this energy bonanza, we invented tools to separate the starchy center from the outer hull, leaving pure starch. Since starch digestion starts in the mouth by an enzyme in saliva, most is completely digested by the time it gets to the small intestine, where the small, powerful sugars rapidly enter the bloodstream.

The resulting stress is directly linked to obesity and a raft of degenerative disorders. Remember that energy (calories) in excess of metabolic need must be stored. If glycogen stores are already full (as is always the case in a sedentary person) these calories MUST be converted to fat.

> Excess calories do not evaporate. They must be stored as glycogen or fat.

Hopefully, you just got another connection between exercise and body composition. Yes, it is true that regular exercise will deplete glycogen stores in the liver and muscles, thereby allowing for the conversion of excess calories to those storage sites. But considering the massive amount of grain that Americans are consuming today, plus all the added sugar, you would have to exercise vigorously for many hours a day to prevent a lot of this from ending up on your thighs, abdomen or butt.

Then there is the metabolic stress. In addition to the excess amount of starch-derived glucose, refined grain products (anything made with flour) deliver simple sugars rapidly into a system that was designed for the slow-release energy of plants.

What about grains consumed whole, like long-grain brown rice, buckwheat, quinoa and amaranth?

Because grains in their whole natural state require a great deal more chewing and digestion compared to ground grain products, they are a far healthier choice.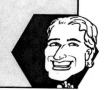

Grinding and refining seem to be the issue. Historically, portability and convenience were major factors, but there is also the modern obsession with whiteness, and the illusion of purity. White flour, white rice, white starchy corn. Barley is a good example of how the degree of refining affects the metabolic value of the food. In order to eat barley (one of the oldest grains) you have to remove the hull. This produces a product called "hulled barley," barley "groats," or "Scotch barley," in which the bran and the germ are intact.

Unfortunately, the vast majority of barley consumed today is "pearled" barley in which the hull and the bran are removed and the resulting material is further polished to create a pure white product that cooks fast and is easy to chew. Therein lies the problem.

Because of the well-understood value of whole grains,[14] I am at odds with Paleo-diet promoters and numerous nutrition "gurus" who believe that grains are akin to poison. There is a world of difference between a commercial breakfast cereal and a bowl of buckwheat groats. Buckwheat and other whole grains have been extensively studied for their ability to reduce risk for cardiovascular disease and Type 2 diabetes.[15,16,17]

Now, what about wheat?

The human brain is wired for black and white decisions, because those are fast and easy; good for survival. But when it comes to complex issues, all-or-nothing thinking can lead to confusion and error. We've seen this with soy, and I think the same thing is happening today with corn and wheat.

There are legitimate and important issues concerning both grains. I think the issues of genetic modification (GMO) are very real and pressing since GMO wheat was approved for planting in 2012. At the very least, a moratorium on further GMO development would allow for a careful scientific review. Monsanto should be forced to demonstrate safety and vastly improved yields, when so far (with GMO corn and soy) they have only demonstrated vastly improved profits.

Beyond GMO, of course, there are the issues of gluten allergy, gluten sensitivity and celiac disease. First, let's discuss celiac disease, which is a genetic disease caused by a number of gene variants with designations like DQ2.5 and DQ8, that reside on chromosome 6.

Most people with celiac disease inherit only one copy of the DQ2.5 gene variant. They may be generally symptom free, but feel bad when they eat a lot of wheat. Others inherit the gene from both parents, and exposure to gluten can produce serious and severe complications.

That's because the protein known as alpha gliadin (aka gluten) triggers an autoimmune reaction that damages the small intestine. Gluten is found in wheat and wheat subspecies including spelt, semolina and durum, and related species such as barley, rye, triticale and Khorasan wheat (also known as Kamut). Gluten is not found in oats, but may be present since that grain is often milled on equipment that is also used for wheat.

Prevalence of Celiac Disease in North America

If you count cases confirmed by colonoscopy and biopsy, incidence is estimated at 1 in 1,750. But if you count people who feel better when they stop eating wheat, the number increases to about 1 in 100.

What about gluten "intolerance" & wheat allergy?

This is where it gets tricky. I spent 6 years studying food allergy and intolerance. My lab developed the first reliable blood test known as the Food Immune Complex Assay or FICA. So I can say with confidence that many people do not do well with wheat, for a variety of reasons. Today, doctors have a variety of tests to evaluate wheat allergy, and "intolerance," which is more of a digestion issue.

On the allergy side, you have "fixed" allergies, mediated by Immunoglobulin E (IgE) which can be serious. These are the rush-the-patient-to-the-hospital reactions (called anaphylaxis) where the lips and throat swell. Wheat is NOT a common IgE allergy. More often, it is mediated by IgG, and this produces less severe symptoms like gastrointestinal discomfort, headache, and constipation/diarrhea. Importantly, IgG reactions can usually be "cleared" either by avoiding wheat or in many cases by including wheat infrequently (the rotation diet strategy).

IgG reactions are also dose related. If your doctor has diagnosed an IgG mediated wheat allergy, he or she will probably advise you to avoid wheat or use a rotation diet plan. But it is very unlikely that they will ask you to examine every label of every product and assiduously avoid any molecule of any substance that could have possibly had contact with wheat.

Years ago when the USDA was drafting warning guidelines for food allergens, the joke among my colleagues was that all food products should carry the statement:

> **WARNING:** this product was produced on a planet where wheat and soy are grown.

NOTE: I am not being glib about the reality of food allergy. Only asking for sanity and the understanding that (unless you have celiac disease) everything is dose related. With true celiac disease, small amounts can cause symptoms. But the rest of us should not worry if the knife that sliced our salmon in the kitchen of our favorite restaurant had previously been used to slice bread.

A systematic review published in 2008 concluded that consumption of less than 10 mg of gluten per day is unlikely to cause harm, even in celiac patients.[18]

The Bottom Line on Grain

Eat a wide variety of natural whole grains, focusing on ancient species such as long grain brown rice, wild rice, quinoa, amaranth and buckwheat.

Try avoiding foods made with flour. People who do this usually report a significant improvement in their health, which doesn't necessarily mean they were allergic to wheat. Eliminating flour products also removes most high-carbohydrate (often high-sugar) foods that cause metabolic stress.

Since most food allergens are proteins (casein in milk, gluten in wheat, albumin in eggs) you can reduce the allergy potential of any meal by optimizing digestion. Eat slowly and chew well. If you still have digestive problems, consider using a comprehensive enzyme with high potency protease (protein-digesting) enzymes.

If no one in your family has celiac disease, it is unlikely that you do. On the other hand, if celiac runs in your family, you would be wise to avoid gluten as much as possible even if you currently have no symptoms.

If you want to unmask a hidden problem with wheat (allergy or intolerance) avoid all products made with wheat, (including spelt, semolina and durum) as well as barley, rye, triticale and Kamut for two weeks. Then, consume a moderate amount of wheat, e.g., two slices of bread or a plate of pasta as part of a simple meal. In other words, you want to consume a small number of foods including wheat, in order to create a "normal" challenge. Go about your day as you normally would, checking in every 30 minutes or so to note how you feel.

Be especially watchful for feelings of profound fatigue, intestinal symptoms (pain, bloating), headache, itching or a visible rash.

Does modern wheat contain more gluten than ancient wheat?

Yes. Through centuries of selective breeding, farmers have been able to alter the gluten content of wheat in order to create the enormous variety of wheat flours available today. Gluten produces a "tough" flour that, when made into dough, confers a stretchiness that is great for making bread. Thus some bread flours have a gluten content close to 45%. Next in gluten content are flours made from hard wheat with gluten levels of 12.5-13.5%. All-purpose flour contains about 10-12% gluten and is actually a mix of high and low gluten wheat flours. Pastry flour contains about 9-10% gluten, and lastly, cake flour (made from soft wheat) is only about 7-9% gluten. Flour high in gluten content doesn't make very good cakes as the cake would lose its soft, crumbly characteristics. To make good angel food cake, for example, requires flour with less than 5% gluten.

3. DAIRY PRODUCTS

Milk was a key contributor to improving nutrition and food security for early humans. It provided protein, essential fats, vitamins, minerals and a raft of immune-support compounds like colostrum, lactalbumin and lactoferrin. Evidence suggests that the milk of domesticated animals like sheep, goats and yaks has been consumed for at least 12,000 years.

About that time, Neolithic herdsmen of Central Asia found that the natural enzymes in the carrying containers (animal stomachs) curdled the milk, essentially making yogurt. This kept the milk from spoiling and made it more transportable. Much later, fermented milk products would be a major fuel for the armies of the Roman and Mongolian Empires. Thus the practice of fermenting or culturing dairy products became widespread throughout Europe, the Middle East and Asia.

So what's all the fuss about?

The dairy controversy, once again, stems from the limited attention span of modern men and women. We are so busy, our brains are constantly looking for black and white issues. It is easy (and fast) to say that dairy is poison, as suggested by a number of books, websites and a popular movie. It takes time to survey the scientific literature and arrive at a more accurate conclusion. Let me summarize what we know. I'll carefully reference my statements so you can study the issue further.

There are 4 main issues:
  A. The ethics of factory farming
  B. The way milk is processed (e.g., pasteurization, homogenization)
  C. Lactose; the predominate sugar in milk.
  D. Casein—one of the proteins in milk—being particularly difficult to digest.

A. ETHICS

Very few people today wake up in the morning to go out and milk the family cow. In modern "factory dairies," cows are kept indoors, injected with hormones to increase milk production, fed corn (an unnatural diet for a ruminant) and treated with antibiotics to combat diseases produced by the poor living conditions.

Thus, once again, it is important to support organic farming. For Natalie and me, this not only means hormone and anti-biotic-free, it means humane treatment and pasture raised. Check your source of milk, and buy local as much as possible.

B. PROCESSING

Pasteurization

To kill the microbes that thrive in milk, most milk sold in North America is pasteurized by heating it to 71.7°C (161°F) for 15 to 20 seconds. Raw-milk enthusiasts claim that this reduces the nutritional value of the milk, and causes milk allergy and lactose intolerance. I could find no evidence that any of that is true. Pasteurization, after all, has no effect on the lactose or casein component of the milk, and while pasteurization does reduce levels of some vitamins (like C and folic acid), milk is not a significant source of these nutrients in the first place.[19] Still, raw milk "wars" have been raging for nearly half a century. The US Centers for Disease Control (CDC) posts a long list of possible contaminants, including bacteria, viruses, and parasites, and states: "From 1998 through 2009, 93 outbreaks due to consumption of raw milk or raw milk products were reported to CDC. These resulted in 1,837 illnesses, 195 hospitalizations, and 2 deaths."[20]

To many people, this is a reasonable risk. Reasonable yes, but unnecessary. My 6 incredibly healthy children (including two adopted from Ethiopia) have consumed a moderate amount of pasteurized milk and cheese. They tend to consume less milk as they enter adulthood—which is a good thing—considering milk intolerance and allergy increase with advancing age.

Homogenization

This is a different story. As I see it, pasteurization is intended to protect the consumer. Homogenization only helps the producers and sellers. In raw milk, the butterfat (cream) is in large globules that tend to rise to the top of the container. Homogenization breaks these into smaller globules that remain distributed throughout the milk, which extends shelf life.

Is homogenization bad for you? For decades, raw milk enthusiasts have looked for evidence that reducing the particle size of butterfat contributes to atherosclerosis, allergy or other health risks. So far, however, homogenization has not been shown to be a problem.[21],[22] What's more, the issue disappears if you use fat-free or fat-reduced milk.

C. LACTOSE

Babies produce an enzyme (lactase) which splits milk sugar (lactose) into two monosaccharides, glucose and galactose. Some people keep producing this enzyme into adulthood. Those who do not continue making lactase become, to varying degrees, lactose intolerant. Because undigested lactose ferments, producing a number of gasses, this can cause symptoms including abdominal bloating and cramps, flatulence, and diarrhea.

In a way, lactose intolerance is inherited, insofar as its prevalence depends on your genetics. People of European descent have a lower incidence of lactose intolerance because of a genetic history of dairy farming. In populations with no history of dairy farming, including most Asians and African Americans, 70% to 90% of the adult population may be affected. Moreover, most everyone produces less lactase as they get older. This is because the cells that produce lactase reside on the surface of the small intestine, and these cells are damaged by a host of factors, including wear and tear, infection, antibiotics, and a variety of drugs.

People who are lactose intolerant should probably not drink regular milk. But lactose-free milk is available in grocery stores throughout North America. **In addition, lactase enzyme drops are available that can be added to milk to reduce or eliminate the lactose.**

Fermenting milk with the beneficial bacteria lactobacillus acidophilus is yet another way for lactase-deficient people to enjoy dairy products. A wide variety of "cultured" dairy products are available and there is plenty of evidence that these products, ranging from "acidophilus milk" to yogurt and kefir, are easier to digest for most people.

Cheese is also easier to digest for people with lactose intolerance. This is because cheese (with the exception of soft cheeses like ricotta) is naturally low in lactose. Moreover, as cheese ages and loses moisture, lactose levels fall even further.

D. MILK PROTEIN ALLERGY (MPA)

Unlike lactose intolerance, which results from the lack of a specific digestive enzyme, milk protein allergy is caused by the protein itself. You can have plenty of lactase and still have MPA, because casein (the primary culprit) resists digestion.

NOTE: When you think of protein, I want you to think of structures. Every structure in the human body is comprised of protein, and protein itself is structural, in that its constituent amino acids form complex chains that fold, interlace and bind other molecules.

Casein exists in milk in complex structures containing hundreds of amino acids bound with calcium and phosphorus. When milk is consumed, the casein interacts with stomach acid to form a gel. In terms of nutrition, this is a good thing, because that gel behaves like a time-release protein source. Bodybuilders often consume pure casein in order to maximize amino acid availability to working muscles.

But this slow-digesting characteristic of casein can also contribute to food allergy. Remember that food allergy is most frequently due to the immune system reacting to a foreign protein. Thus proteins that are hard to digest (e.g., gluten, casein) tend to be the most allergenic. Your body likes its protein delivered as fully-digested amino acids or very small peptides. Intact proteins from another species (e.g., a cow) are unwelcome in your bloodstream, and set off an immune reaction known as allergy.

Estimates are that 1% to 10% of babies in the Western world have MPA.[23],[24] Most "outgrow" this allergy (in other words, their digestive tract becomes competent at digesting casein) by early childhood,[25] but some do not, and continue to have symptoms into adulthood.

However, MPA is not just a "digestion thing." It is equally an "immune system thing," because people with allergy to milk tend to have other allergies. It is not unlikely for a milk-protein allergy to reappear later in life, either as a result of impaired digestion, a defect in the barrier mechanism of the gut, or a combination of factors.

Again, allergy to milk protein can be mediated by IgE or IgG, determined by medical tests. Those with high levels of IgE antibodies are usually considered truly allergic, while elevations of IgG can indicate a milk-protein intolerance. The difference is an important one, since "true" MPA (with high levels of IgE antibodies) typically produce more serious symptoms that may include impaired breathing and (rarely) anaphylaxis, a rapidly progressing, life-threatening reaction.

As with gluten, milk-protein intolerance tends to be dose related. I'm 65 years old, come from dairy-farming ancestors, have stellar digestion, but would not do well with a cherry cheesecake or a full glass of milk.

Factory farming, allergy and intolerance... why bother eating dairy products?

Dairy Foods Support Anabolic (Build/Repair) Metabolism

Studies with both men and women have shown that dairy foods support muscle mass and bone strength better than equal amounts of other high-protein foods.[26],[27]

Cultured Dairy Provides Valuable Probiotics

Here's a quote from a leading study published in Applied Microbiology and Biotechnology.

"Probiotics have a number of beneficial health effects in humans, such as reducing lactose intolerance symptoms

and enhancing the bioavailability of nutrients. Probiotics help regulate intestinal microflora and immunomodulatory properties. Probiotics also decrease the prevalence of allergies in susceptible individuals, inhibit the inflammatory responses in the gut, and have antagonistic effects against intestinal and food-borne pathogens.[28]

Cultured dairy foods have also been found to reduce dental plaque and help prevent cavities.[29] I'm including all of this information to balance out the "anti-dairy" material that continues to proliferate on the Internet. Posters appear claiming that the calcium in milk is not absorbable, that everyone is lactose intolerant or allergic and that dairy foods increase risk for cancer and heart disease. All of these statements are either unproven or patently false.

Opinion One Internet site states: *"The animal protein, fat, and cholesterol (even nonfat/skim milk contains cholesterol) all contribute to heart disease, certain cancers, diabetes, and other major chronic disease."*[30]

Evidence A peer-reviewed biomedical journal states: *"The observational evidence does not support the hypothesis that dairy fat or high-fat dairy foods contribute to obesity or cardiometabolic risk, and suggests that high-fat dairy consumption within typical dietary patterns is inversely associated with obesity risk."*[31]

Want more ammunition to **debunk dairyphobia?** There's plenty. In contrast to the book, The China Study, a meta-analysis of 18 published studies—including more than a million participants—found that milk and total dairy consumption was associated with reduced risk for breast cancer. Using the most stringent statistical criteria, the reduced risk was strongly associated with total dairy, while milk consumption was only somewhat associated with reduced incidence of breast cancer. The study concluded that: *"Findings of the present meta-analysis indicate that increased consumption of total dairy food...may be associated with a reduced risk of breast cancer."*[32]

I am not suggesting that women run out and start quaffing dairy products, but this study (which took place at the Department of Nutrition and Food Hygiene, Soochow University, Suzhou, China) casts a great deal of doubt on any claim that dairy somehow increases risk for breast cancer.

Studies in China have also found an association between consumption of low-fat milk and yogurt with higher levels of adiponectin, one of the primary metabolic modifiers that we will discuss in Chapter 8.
This in turn reduces risk for diabetes and obesity.[33]

The Bottom Line on Dairy

For those who are not lactose intolerant or allergic to milk, dairy products can be an important source of protein, vitamins, minerals essential fats and beneficial probiotics. We've been talking a lot about how human physiology adapts to changes in diet and the environment. Dairy products have been consumed by about 450 generations, which in the span of human history is not that long, but it is sufficient for large numbers of humans – those with a genetic history of dairy farming – to develop the ability to digest and use the cornucopia of nutrients provided by dairy foods.

Once again, it comes down to a metabolic issue. If you consume dairy products and have no symptoms, it is likely due to your body's production of lactase, and/or your selection of low-lactose products like yogurt and aged cheese. I rarely consume cow's milk, but enjoy whey, cheese and unsweetened yogurt. Natalie (though also descended from traditionally dairy-herding ancestors) has a more sensitive GI tract. She limits her dairy to goat's milk yogurt (easier to digest, available from grass-fed, organic sources) and cheese made from the milk of goats or sheep.

4. A MEATY ISSUE

Our ancestors ate wild game whenever they could. So do hunter/gatherers today. The difference, however, between wild meat and domesticated beef is staggering. A study of 15 species of African animals showed a fat content of just 3.9%. In contrast, thanks to modern breeding and feeding practices, beef today contains 20% to 35% fat.

Not only is this meat marbled with fat, nearly every gram of it is nonessential, artery-clogging fat. Compare that with wild game, which is low in total and saturated fat and relatively rich in omega-3 fatty acids. In fact, research shows that lean meat from wild game actually lowers cholesterol levels and contributes significant amounts of protein, essential fats, iron, zinc, and vitamin B12.[34]

Modern meat is also laced with antibiotics and hormones that are required to keep animals alive in fetid feedlot conditions. This has resulted in an astounding increase in diseased animals going to market.

There are numerous reasons to purchase organically-raised meat. Recent studies with the elderly show an increase in mortality related to high meat consumption.[35] I believe this is related, not to the protein (as some vegetarians speculate) but to the fat content of modern meat, as well as the hormones, antibiotics and toxins.

Following is a list of "wild" and/or naturally-raised meat sources:

- Bison
- Venison
- Antelope
- Alligator
- Elk
- Caribou
- Emu
- Grass-fed, organic beef
- Grass-fed lamb
- Goat
- Moose
- Rabbit
- Frog legs
- Wild boar
- Pheasant
- Quail
- Organic duck
- Organic goose
- Partridge
- Ostrich
- Kangaroo
- Rattlesnake
- Turtle
- Yak

NOTE: Meat Preparation is important

We know that charbroiled or grilled meat carries a significant health risk as polycyclic aromatic hydrocarbons (PAHs) deposit on the meat from the charcoal, wood or gas flames. And no matter what kind of meat you consume, the longer you cook it, the greater are the heath risks. Studies suggest, in fact, that the association of meat eating with increased cancer risk disappears if you limit your cooking time. People who eat their meat cooked rare or medium rare do not appear to have increased risk for cancer.[36,37,38,39]

5. CHICKEN OR THE EGG?

Hopefully, you're getting the drift in this chapter that animals raised in their natural environment, eating their natural diet are far better for you than factory-farmed animals. This is certainly true for chickens where commercial birds are kept in "cubby cages," too small for the chicken to even turn around, let alone spread her wings. These massive, inhumane assembly-line operations grow chickens under intense artificial light, feed them drug-laced unnatural diets designed not to nourish the birds but to produce rapid growth and deliver the taste that consumers have come to expect; soft (because the meat is mostly fat) and sweet (because their feed is mostly corn and soy).

Chickens kept in these conditions are susceptible to multiple infections and these microbes (E. coli and salmonella) can remain in the meat. Thus, each year in the US alone, contaminated chicken kills approximately 1,000 people and sickens thousands more.[40] Recent studies have found that about 30% of chicken is contaminated with salmonella and over 60% with a related fecal bacteria known as campylobacter.[41,42]

Fortunately, organically-raised chicken is widely available in health food and grocery stores. Even better, support your local poultry farmers, food co-ops and farmer's markets.

What about eggs?

Eggs are a great source of protein, essential fats, minerals (especially sulfur), B vitamins, choline, folic acid and vitamins A, D and E. But please support local, free-range egg producers. At the grocery store, egg carton labels can be confusing.

Cage Free = Eggs from hens that are housed inside a building without being confined to cages. While that sounds more humane, the hens may still be in terribly crowded conditions, and their beaks are usually trimmed to prevent pecking at themselves and others. Many believe beak-trimming is a source of chronic pain for the hens.

Free Range = Suggests that the hens are free to roam around a pasture, but that is rarely the case. "Free range" only means that the door to the facility is open, giving the chicken access to an outdoor area.

Certified Organic = Hens are fed an organic, all-vegetarian diet free of hormones, antibiotics and pesticides, as required by the U.S. Department of Agriculture's National Organic Program.

Vegetarian = Simply means that the hens are fed a grain-based diet free of any animal products. In reality, of course, chickens are not vegetarians. They naturally eat bugs, grubs, worms, grains, grasses and whatever they can scratch from the ground.

I prefer to buy eggs from a neighbor, co-op or farmer's market, where the hens live naturally. Of course, in some areas, where predators are a problem, the chickens are housed in large cages that are placed in the pasture or field, and moved around to enable the birds to eat what birds are supposed to eat.

And yes, compared to conventional egg farms, hens that are allowed to peck on pasture are healthier and produce more nutritious eggs, with higher levels of Vitamin A, omega-3 fatty acids, vitamin E and beta carotene.[43]

NOTE: Adequate cooking of eggs is necessary to kill potential salmonella organisms. On the other hand, eggs should not be overcooked or burned, as we explained in Chapter 5. Overcooking proteins can create toxins known as AGEs (Advanced Glycation Endproducts). Avoid breakfast buffets where the eggs have been heating (and glycating) for hours.

The startling increase in fatty-liver disease that physicians are seeing today has set off an alarm in the research community. Fingers are pointing to the increased consumption of fructose and other sugars, as well as alcohol and the highly processed fats found in junk food. I am sure those contribute to the epidemic. But I also know from diet surveys that most people are deficient in choline, which is essential for removing fat from the liver. Egg-yolk-phobia, and the admonition against eating organ meats may be contributing to fatty-liver disease, since these are by far the best dietary sources of choline. If you are not eating eggs or liver, be sure to take a choline supplement. I recommend at least 500 mg per day.

Organically-raised chicken and eggs coming from your neighborhood farmer's market are your best bet...

6. FISH

For Natalie and me, wild-caught fish is a major protein source. Fish is a nutrition powerhouse, being the best source of omega-3 fatty acids EPA and DHA, as well as complete protein, the entire range of B vitamins, a variety of minerals, and vitamins E and D. Research has shown that regular consumption of fish reduces risk for cardiovascular disease (heart attack, stroke, poor circulation and abnormal clotting), and that these benefits outweigh the potential risk of ingesting toxins such as mercury and PCBs.[44,45]

To minimize the pollution risks, we buy only ocean-caught fish, and focus on oil-rich fish from northern seas, such as Alaskan salmon, snapper, sardines, herring and mackerel. Larger fish at the top of the food chain tend to bio-accumulate toxins, so we tend to avoid swordfish, shark, tuna and Chilean sea bass.

Dealing with Mercury

Consuming 6 to 10 servings of fish per week, doctors and researchers have wondered why my mercury levels are extremely low. I attribute this to high consumption of detox nutrients like selenium and zinc, as well as ingestion of glutathione-stimulating compounds like N-acetyl cysteine (NAC) and whey protein.[46] The glutathione detox pathway is probably the most capable of removing mercury from the body.

In addition, I have been drinking aloe vera for more than 20 years. The terminal end of the aloe polysaccharide is mannose, which appears to bind nicely with mercury, facilitating its removal through the urine and GI tract.

7. THE VEGETARIAN/VEGAN ISSUE

There are many arguments for a vegetarian diet, including ethical and religious beliefs. But the health arguments are usually based on faulty comparisons of vegetarians, who are generally very health-conscious, to the general population consisting mainly of sedentary, overweight people who eat large quantities of junk food.

There is no doubt that a diet of whole, unprocessed plant foods can significantly improve the health of people who were formerly eating a low-nutrient, highly processed, factory-farmed, corn-fed, hormone- and antibiotic-laced Western diet. But the health gains claimed by vegetarians are due just as much to what these folks stopped eating. The argument against moderate consumption of game and/or organically–raised meat is weak, and the argument against eating fish is nonexistent. That is why vegetarian websites and the movie Forks Over Knives pretty much avoid the fish issue. It doesn't fit into their all-or-nothing argument.

The oft-cited example of Norway in WWII is a vegetarian myth. When the Nazis invaded—so the story goes—they took all the livestock to feed German troops. Then, from 1939 to 1945, deaths from cardiovascular disease (CVD) dropped. The assumption is that Norwegians resorted to a plant-based, dairy-less diet, and that produced a rapid drop in CVD. What really happened was that the Norwegians made a number of important adjustments. Published records show that consumption of sugar, butter and margarine dropped dramatically, while (as you would expect) fish consumption doubled![47] They also became very resourceful, eating wild birds (even seagulls) and processing fish roe to make flour. This, together with a 20% reduction in calories, is the more likely explanation for the reduced rate of cardiovascular disease in that period.

But vegetarians live longer, don't they?

Not really. A study of Seventh Day Adventists showed longevity increases of 7.28 years in men and 4.42 years in women.[48] But this, like the majority of similar comparisons, is inconclusive, for the obvious reason that it compared the health and mortality statistics of the average American with people who are not only vegetarian, but who follow a healthy lifestyle free of tobacco and alcohol. Moreover, Seventh Day Adventists strongly favor prevention over prescription drug use, while the average 65 year-old American is on 6 prescription drugs. Prescription drugs, taken as directed, are the fourth leading cause of death in North America.[49]

What happens when you look at the health and mortality stats of **" c o n s c i o u s   o m n i v o r e s ? "** These are people who consume a highly varied natural-foods diet, together with a wide variety of protein from wild-caught ocean fish, eggs from pasture-raised, organically-fed chickens, grass-fed, hormone- and antibiotic–free beef, wild game and organic poultry.

The problem is that these people are difficult to study. They're not concentrated in any one location, nor are they found in a single religious, social or cultural niche. Thus the research has not been done. The closest we get are studies with Mediterranean populations, and there we find stats as good or better than American vegetarians.[50]

What about Vegans?

Longevity and health stats for vegans (vegetarians who also avoid eggs and dairy products) are hard to come by, but it is unlikely that they are any better than what has been compiled for vegetarians. This is not going to make me very popular with my vegan friends, but let's take a look at an important analysis published in the *American Journal of Clinical Nutrition*, comparing the health and mortality stats for 76,172 men and women.[51]

Compared with regular meat eaters, mortality from cardiovascular disease was:

* 20% lower in occasional meat eaters
* 34% lower in people who ate fish but not meat
* 34% lower in lacto-ovo vegetarians (vegetarians consuming dairy and eggs)
* 26% lower in vegans

This strongly suggests that those consuming fish, dairy and eggs fared better than vegans. What about other health claims made for a vegetarian diet? This detailed analysis showed no significant differences between vegetarians and nonvegetarians in mortality from cerebrovascular disease, stomach cancer, colorectal cancer, lung cancer, breast cancer, prostate cancer, or all other causes combined.

Please understand that I have always emphasized the importance of eating a wide variety of vegetables, fruits, legumes and whole ancient grains (in that order). I was a vegetarian for seven years, and perhaps the most important thing I learned was how to prepare vegetarian dishes, so that I never fell into the health-killing trap known as the Standard American Diet.

Natalie and I are "conscious omnivores." That is how I raised my six remarkably healthy kids, and there is plenty of research to support this approach. I appreciate the passion of those who promote a vegetarian, vegan or raw-vegan diet. But very often, these promotions are more romantic than scientific. Claims, for example, that the vegan diet is more "natural" ignore the inconvenient fact that in the history of mankind, there has never been a voluntarily vegan society. In other words, wherever there were animals, fish or fowl, humans ate them and in fact relied on them to survive.

There are, of course cultures in which vegetarianism is based on a religious and/or ethical choice. And as far as I am concerned, there is no argument against that. You simply cannot tell someone that their beliefs are groundless. But virtually all the scientific evidence that is used to promote a vegetarian diet falls apart upon close examination.

The Conscious Omnivore diet

Humans are omnivores. We have large canine teeth and a digestive system with the capacity to extract nutrients from a wide variety of plants, animals, fowl and fish. We cannot create energy from the sun, so we eat plants that do. We cannot gain nourishment from grass or other high-cellulose plants, so we eat the animals that do.

If there is one principle that stands out from the study of human nutrition, it is the need for variety. If you decide to be a vegetarian, do not become a soyatarian. If you decide to be vegan, you will need to pay special attention to preparing a range of beans, grains, seeds and nuts to optimize digestion and protein bioavailability. Long ago, our ancestors learned that soaking, sprouting and fermenting these foods increased their biological value.

"Conscious" not only applies to the selection of whole natural foods, but to the conditions in which the food is grown, raised, and processed. It may take longer to shop at a farmer's market. Organic food is more expensive. But these are important choices, and when we "vote with our wallets," we support the men and women in our community who have a direct link to the rivers, the soil and the sun.

ⓘ
Summary

1. Erroneous or bizarre information posted on the internet is called webaloney. Help stamp out webaloney (and save the internet):
    A. Check the validity of any information before forwarding or posting.
    B. Challenge those who post health information to provide references, preferably to published biomedical literature.

2. If there is one principle that stands out from the study of human nutrition, it is the need for variety.

3. Soy foods are healthful when used as part of a highly varied natural foods diet. They should not be the predominant or sole source of protein.

4. While it is true that humans have only been consuming grain for 12,000 years, that's more than 600 generations; certainly enough time for most people to benefit from these important foods.

5. When you think of the word, "grain," put the word "whole" in front of it. Whole grains, especially the ancient species such as quinoa, buckwheat, amaranth, wild rice and long-grain brown rice, are gluten free, and provide a wide range of health benefits, including reduced risk for diabetes.

6. There are three distinct problems associated with wheat and other gluten grains.
    A. Celiac disease
    B. Allergy, characterized by high levels of antibodies to gluten
    C. Intolerance, due to poor digestion, GI disease or aging

7. Cultured/fermented dairy products are much easier to digest compared to whole milk and are a good source of protein, probiotics, vitamins and minerals. These include yogurt, kefir, buttermilk and cultured cottage cheese.

8. A Vegetarian diet can be extremely healthful, but there is no scientific consensus regarding claims for reduced morbidity and mortality compared to what can be termed a "conscious omnivore" diet.

Endnotes

1 Clawson GA. Protease inhibitors and carcinogenesis: a review. Cancer Invest. 1996;14(6):597-608.

2 Pan Y, Anthony M, Clarkson TB. Effect of estradiol and soy phytoestrogens on choline acetyltransferase and nerve growth factor mRNAs in the frontal cortex and hippocampus of female rats. Proc Soc Exp Biol Med. 1999 Jun;221(2):118-25.

3 Lephart ED, Thompson JM, Setchell KD, Adlercreutz H, Weber KS. Phytoestrogens decrease brain calcium-binding proteins but do not alter hypothalamic androgen metabolizing enzymes in adult male rats. Brain Res 2000 Mar 17;859(1):123-31

4 White LR, Petrovich H, Ross GW, Masaki KH, Association of mid-life consumption of tofu with late life cognitive impairment and dementia: the Honolulu-Asia Aging Study. Fifth International Conference on Alzheimer's Disease, #487, 27 July 1996, Osaka, Japan.

5 2. White LR, Petrovitch H, Ross GW, Masaki KH, Hardman J, Nelson J, Davis D, Markesbery W, Brain aging and midlife tofu consumption. J Am Coll Nutr 2000 Apr;19(2):242-55.

6 Soy Infant Formula Could Be Harmful to Infants: Groups Want it Pulled. Nutrition Week, Dec 10, 1999;29(46):1-2.

7 Setchell KD, Zimmer-Nechemias L, Cai J, Heubi JE, Exposure of infants to phyto-oestrogens from soy-based infant formula. Lancet 1997 Jul 5;350(9070):23-27.

8 Miyagi Y, Shinjo S, Nishida R, Miyagi C, Takamatsu K, Yamamoto T, Yamamoto S. Trypsin inhibitor activity in commercial soybean products in Japan. J Nutr Sci Vitaminol. 1997 Oct;43(5):575-80

9 Divi RL, Chang HC, Doerge DR, Anti-thyroid isoflavones from soybean: isolation, characterization, and mechanisms of action.Biochem Pharmacol 1997 Nov 15;54(10):1087-96.

10 Shepard TH. Soybean Goiter. New Eng J Med 1960; 262;1099-1103

11 REF: de Kleijn MJ, van der Schouw YT, Wilson PW, Adlercreutz H, Mazur W, Grobbee DE, et al. Intake of dietary phytoestrogens is low in postmenopausal women in the United States: the Framingham study. J Nutr. 2001;131:1826–32.

12 Boucher BA, Cotterchio M, Anderson LN, et al. Use of isoflavone supplements is associated with reduced postmenopausal breast cancer risk. International Journal of Cancer. 15 March 2013; Volume 132, Issue 6, pages 1439–1450.

13   Agriculture Fact Book | Chapter 2, Profiling Food Consumption in America. USDA's Center for Nutrition Policy and Promotion; USDA's Economic Research Service. 2011.

14   Granfeldt Y, Eliasson AC, Björck I. An examination of the possibility of lowering the glycemic index of oat and barley flakes by minimal processing. J Nutr. 2000 Sep;130(9):2207-14.

15   Kim J, Shin J, Lee S. Cardioprotective effects of diet with different grains on lipid profiles and antioxidative system in obesity-induced rats. Int J Vitam Nutr Res. 2012 Apr;82(2):85-93

16   Sharafetdinov KhKh, Gapparov MM, Plotnikova OA, Zykina VV, Shlelenko LA, Tiurina OE, Rabotkin IuV. Influence of breads with use of barley, buckwheat and oat flours and barley flakes on postprandial glycaemia in patients with type 2 diabetes mellitus. Vopr Pitan. 2009;78(4):40-6.

17   Venn BJ, Mann JI. Cereal grains, legumes and diabetes. Eur J Clin Nutr. 2004 Nov;58(11):1443-61.

18   Akobeng AK, Thomas AG (June 2008). "Systematic review: tolerable amount of gluten for people with coeliac disease". Aliment. Pharmacol. Ther. 27 (11): 1044–52.

19   Macdonald LE, Brett J, Kelton D, Majowicz SE, Snedeker K, Sargeant JM.A systematic review and meta-analysis of the effects of pasteurization on milk vitamins, and evidence for raw milk consumption and other health-related outcomes. J Food Prot. 2011 Nov;74(11):1814-32.

20   http://www.cdc.gov/foodsafety/rawmilk/raw-milk-questions-and-answers.html accessed 11/17/12

21   Clifford AJ, Ho CY, Swenerton H.Homogenized bovine milk xanthine oxidase: a critique of the hypothesis relating to plasmalogen depletion and cardiovascular disease. Am J Clin Nutr. 1983 Aug;38(2):327-32.

22   Paajanen L, Tuure T, Poussa T, Korpela R.No difference in symptoms during challenges with homogenized and unhomogenized cow's milk in subjects with subjective hypersensitivity to homogenized milk. J Dairy Res. 2003 May;70(2):175-9.

23   Constantinide P, Trandafir LM, Burlea M. The role of specific IgE to evolution and prognosis of cow's milk protein allergies in children. Rev Med Chir Soc Med Nat Iasi. 2011 Oct-Dec;115(4):1012-7.

24   Brand PL, Rijk-van Gent H. Cow's milk allergy in infants: new insights. Ned Tijdschr Geneeskd. 2011;155(27):A3508.

25   Ahrens B, Lopes de Oliveira LC, Grabenhenrich L, Schulz G, Niggemann B, Wahn U, Beyer K. Individual cow's milk allergens as prognostic markers for tolerance development? Clin Exp Allergy. 2012 Nov;42(11):1630-7.

26   Josse AR, Phillips SM. Impact of milk consumption and resistance training on body composition of female athletes. Med Sport Sci. 2013;59:94-103. doi: 10.1159/000341968. Epub 2012 Oct 15.

27   Hartman JW, Tang JE, Wilkinson SB, Tarnopolsky MA, Lawrence RL, Fullerton AV, Phillips SM. Consumption of fat-free fluid milk after resistance exercise promotes greater lean mass accretion than does consumption of soy or carbohydrate in young, novice, male weightlifters. Am J Clin Nutr. 2007 Aug;86(2):373-81.

28   Tsai YT, Cheng PC, Pan TM. The immunomodulatory effects of lactic acid bacteria for improving immune functions and benefits. Appl Microbiol Biotechnol. 2012 Nov;96(4):853-62.

29   Ravishankar TL, Yadav V, Tangade PS, Tirth A, Chaitra TR. Effect of consuming different dairy products on calcium, phosphorus and pH levels of human dental plaque: a comparative study. Eur Arch Paediatr Dent. 2012 Jun;13(3):144-8.

30   http://www.forksoverknives.com/nutrition-faq/ accessed 11-18-12

31   Kratz M, Baars T, Guyenet S. The relationship between high-fat dairy consumption and obesity, cardiovascular, and metabolic disease. Eur J Nutr. 2012 Jul 19.

32   Dong JY, Zhang L, He K, Qin LQ. Dairy consumption and risk of breast cancer: a meta-analysis of prospective cohort studies. Breast Cancer Res Treat. 2011 May;127(1):23-31.

33   Niu K, Kobayashi Y, Guan L, Monma H, Guo H, Cui Y, Otomo A, Chujo M, Nagatomi R. Low-fat dairy, but not whole-/high-fat dairy, consumption is related with higher serum adiponectin levels in apparently healthy adults. Eur J Nutr. 2012 May 31.

34   Mann N. Dietary lean red meat and human evolution. Eur J Nutr 2000 Apr;39(2):71-9

35   Fortes C, Forastiere F, Farchi S, Rapiti E, Pastori G, Perucci CA. Diet and overall survival in a cohort of very elderly people. Epidemiology. 2000 Jul;11(4):440-5.

36   Figg WD 2nd. How do you want your steak prepared? The impact of meat consumption and preparation on prostate cancer. Cancer Biol Ther. 2012 Oct 1;13(12):1141-2. doi: 10.4161/cbt.21463.

37   Ferguson LR. Meat and cancer. Meat Sci. 2010 Feb;84(2):308-13.

38   Kabat GC, Cross AJ, Park Y, Schatzkin A, Hollenbeck AR, Rohan TE, Sinha R. Meat intake and meat preparation in relation to risk of post-menopausal breast cancer in the NIH-AARP diet and health study. Int J Cancer. 2009 May 15;124(10):2430-5. doi: 10.1002/ijc.24203.

39   Anderson KE, Mongin SJ, Sinha R, Stolzenberg-Solomon R, Gross MD, Ziegler RG, Mabie JE, Risch A, Kazin SS, Church TR. Pancreatic cancer risk: associations with meat-derived carcinogen intake in the Prostate, Lung, Colorectal, and Ovarian Cancer Screening Trial (PLCO) cohort. Mol Carcinog. 2012 Jan;51(1):128-37.

40   Richard Behar and Michael Kramer, Something Smells Fowl. Time, Oct 17, 1994, pg 42. Jane Brody, Personal Health, New York Times Oct 5, 1994.

41   Smith C, JD DeWaal. Playing Chicken: The Human Cost of inadequate regulation of the Poultry Industry. Center for Science in the Public Interest. March, 1996, pg 2.

42   Berrang ME, Buhr RJ, Cason JA. Campylobacter recovery from external and internal organs of commercial broiler carcass prior to scalding. Poult Sci. 2000 Feb;79(2):286-90.

43   http://www.motherearthnews.com/Real-Food/2007-10-01/Tests-Reveal-Healthier-Eggs.aspx#ixzz2Do28iOEF Accessed on 12/1/12

44   Di Minno MN, Tremoli E, Tufano A, Russolillo A, Lupoli R, Di Minno G. Exploring newer cardioprotective strategies: ω-3 fatty acids in perspective. Thromb Haemost. 2010 Oct;104(4):664-80.

45   http://www.hsph.harvard.edu/nutritionsource/what-should-you-eat/fish/

46   Joshi D, Mittal D, Shrivastav S, Shukla S, Srivastav AK.Combined effect of N-acetyl cysteine, zinc, and selenium against chronic dimethylmercury-induced oxidative stress: a biochemical and histopathological approach. Arch Environ Contam Toxicol. 2011 Nov;61(4):558-67

47   Angell-Andersen E, Tretli S, Bjerknesz R, et al. The association between nutritional conditions during World War II and childhood anthropometric variables in the Nordic countries. Annals of Human Biology May-June   2004,   VOL.   31, NO. 3, 342 – 355 Accessed on 11/25, 2012 at: http://www.lorentzcenter.nl/lc/web/2008/319/CD%20LORENTZ%20CENTER%20WORKSHOP/NORDIC%20angell-andersen%20ann%20hum%20biol%202004.pdf

48   Fraser GE, Shavlik DJ. Ten years of life: Is it a matter of choice? Arch Intern Med. 2001 Jul 9;161(13):1645-52.

49 US Department of Health and Human Services /US FDA. Preventable Adverse Drug Reactions: A Focus on Drug Interactions. Accessed 11/25/12 at: http://www.fda.gov/drugs/developmentapprovalprocess/ developmentresources/druginteractionslabeling/ucm110632.htm

50 Sofi F, Cesari F, Abbate R, Gensini GF, Casini A. Adherence to Mediterranean diet and health status: meta-analysis. BMJ. 2008 Sep 11;337:a1344.

51 Key TJ, Fraser GE, Thorogood M, et al. Mortality in vegetarians and non-vegetarians: detailed findings from a collaborative analysis of 5 prospective studies. Am J Clin Nutr. 1999 Sep;70(3 Suppl):516S-24S.

Chapter Seven

Not Eating

Our ancient ancestors, whose bodies we inherited, ate and weighed a good deal less in relation to their size than we do. Over hundreds of thousands of years their desire for food was checked by its scarcity and the effort it took to collect it daily from the countryside. Thereby they set the reference standard for living and eating normally and healthily, not we. We eat as much as we like. No creature has ever been adapted to that.

~ Nobel Prize winner, Hans G. Demelt, University of Washington

The previous 2 chapters have been about what and how to eat. This one is about not eating. Anthropologists tell us that human history was filled with periods of scarcity and famine. Evolutionary biologists note that this would most certainly have an effect on the human genome, meaning that we are designed for periods of scarcity and/or immanent starvation.

What then are we to think about the modern habit of eating three meals plus snacks, 365 days a year, with periodic feasts and frequent overeating? It appears that, once again, we are out of synch with our genes. Some of the consequences are obvious (our expanding waistlines), but others are invisible.

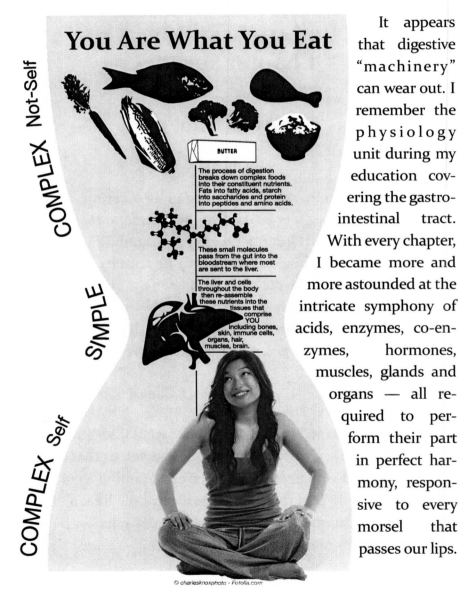

You Are What You Eat

The process of digestion breaks down complex foods into their constituent nutrients. Fats into fatty acids, starch into saccharides and protein into peptides and amino acids.

These small molecules pass from the gut into the bloodstream where most are sent to the liver.

The liver and cells throughout the body then re-assemble these nutrients into the tissues that comprise YOU including bones, skin, immune cells, organs, hair, muscles, brain.

COMPLEX Not-Self

SIMPLE

COMPLEX Self

© charlesknoxphoto - Fotolia.com

It appears that digestive "machinery" can wear out. I remember the physiology unit during my education covering the gastrointestinal tract. With every chapter, I became more and more astounded at the intricate symphony of acids, enzymes, co-enzymes, hormones, muscles, glands and organs — all required to perform their part in perfect harmony, responsive to every morsel that passes our lips.

Overeating taxes the ability of this system to process foreign (not-self) material, essentially to reduce complex foods—in massive molecular structures—down to their constituent small molecular weight compounds so that that your body can then re-assemble these nutrients into the complex structures called self; your bones, blood, heart, skin, hair, brain, and the like.

The greatest burden falls on the pancreas, small intestine, liver and kidneys; and evidence suggests that non-stop eating is contributing to the damage, degeneration and disease associated with these organs.

The good news is that getting back in synch with our genes, and reaping significant metabolic benefits, is rather easy. The process unfolds in a 2-step process.

STEP 1: STOP OVEREATING

I had the opportunity, many years ago, to attend a centennial birthday party. The man who was celebrating his 10th decade of life was Japanese, living in San Francisco. Not only was he independent; he raised a backyard garden, used public transportation to maintain an active social calendar, and cognition testing showed that his memory and information-processing speed was that of a man in his mid 50's.

I asked him for the secret to his remarkable health. He replied, "I eat when I am hungry and I stop eating when my hunger is gone."

Perplexed, I said, "Well, so do I."

"No you don't," he said softly. "You probably eat until you are full. If you are like most people, you sometimes eat until you are stuffed."

My silence indicated agreement.

"Try to be sensitive," he said, "to the point where your hunger is *satisfied*. You will be surprised at how little food that requires. Stop there, even if your tongue wants more. Tell your tongue that if you are truly hungry in a few hours, you can have more to eat."

THUS BEGAN MY HABIT OF CONSCIOUS EATING.

In clinical practice, I saw many clients who would recoil at the thought of depriving themselves of a second helping or a massive dessert. We all carry within us the DNA of starving ancestors, so I was certainly not critical. My approach was more educational. "Digestion," I would say, "is like a chemical fire. Imagine you're on a camping trip and the weather has turned. You're desperate to start a fire. Your cold hands are shaking as you carefully pile some kindling on top of crumpled paper. You are alarmed to see that you only have two matches, so everything has to be timed perfectly. Light the match, the paper ignites, a few twigs catch fire, then a few more. You are just starting to feel the warmth on your face from an ancient survival skill...then your friend throws a huge soggy log on the fire. It sputters, and goes out."

Rarely did I have to explain the metaphor, but I would continue: "**When you overload your digestive 'fire,' it smolders and sputters, leaving undigested food in your GI tract.** It's very warm and moist down there, so this material quickly ferments and putrefies, creating the bloating and discomfort that you noted on your symptom list. And that's only the beginning. These chemical reactions produce toxins that increase your risk of serious intestinal disease, and some are absorbed into your bloodstream creating other problems."

That would usually do it, but some clients would still protest that they had already tried to push themselves away from the table, but to no avail. That's when I would put on my counselor's hat and talk about behavior modification. It's not about *"should"* and *"oughts."* It's not finger-wagging and certainly not about guilt and blame.

Overeating is a *habit*. We have all created the physical and emotional cues that determine our eating habits. And while habits do not change overnight, they can be changed through awareness. After a meal, the only thing you should feel is not hungry. There should be no discomfort whatsoever. No bloating, gas or pain. No having to let your belt out a few notches. Eating slowly is the most important tool. Savor every mouthful. Put your fork down between bites, and don't pick it up until your food has been thoroughly chewed, swallowed and appreciated.

Metabolic Modifiers: In the next chapter, you'll read about compounds that can help you eat less. Some increase your sense of satiety (hunger satisfaction), while others reduce carb cravings.

When you have conquered overeating, you are ready for step 2: Skip a Meal - which requires a short (and fun) physiology lesson.

HOW YOUR BODY WORKS: IT'S ALL ABOUT ENERGY

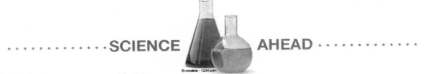

Glycogen and Fat

Since life, until very recently, was fraught with short and sometimes lengthy periods of famine, humans evolved the ability to store energy. For short famines (one to two days), glycogen stores in the liver and muscles work just fine. For longer periods, we survived by burning stored fat.

You'll remember from Chapter 4 that glycogen is a polysaccharide, with more than 20,000 glucose units branched around a core protein.

The liver has an amazing capacity to store glycogen, and the branching structure made it possible for the liver to release multiple glucose units when we were being chased by saber-toothed tigers.

Now, I know what you're thinking: "I thought the liver was responsible for detoxification." True, but detox is only one of about 60 functions performed by this amazing organ. The liver acts as the clearinghouse for nutrient delivery to every cell in the body and plays a critical role in energy metabolism. When blood sugar is low, or we're facing an emergency, it releases glycogen. When blood sugar levels are high, it makes glycogen. If glycogen stores are full, it converts glucose to fat (triglyceride) and ships it off to the bloodstream. When blood triglycerides get too high, the liver ships the fat to your thighs, abdomen or buttocks. In the world of energy management, the liver is command central.

A limited amount of glycogen is also stored in the muscles, including the heart.

During pregnancy, the uterus also stores glycogen to nourish the fetus, and later to fuel contractions during delivery.

♥

The point of this discussion is to introduce you to a metabolic secret, which you may have already guessed. There is an important connection between glycogen and insulin. The muscles and liver release glycogen as needed, to fuel exercise or to maintain glucose levels between meals. Think of it as glucose on demand, when cells are eager for energy. Providing this energy requires very little insulin.

For most people, on the other hand, meals are glucose overload. Cells are resistant to the action of insulin, so the pancreas, desperate to lower blood sugar, produces even more insulin. Elevated blood glucose and elevated insulin then wreak havoc throughout the body and brain.

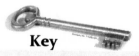

Key

Fortunately, there is another way to quickly dispose of glucose. Your body can convert it to glycogen but only if glycogen stores are low. How do you deplete glycogen stores? Exercise and/or skip a meal.

You're probably also wondering how to increase glycogen capacity to take maximum advantage of this insulin and glucose-lowering strategy. Well, let's see... Glycogen is stored in the liver and muscles. You can't make your liver any bigger, but muscle mass can be increased, and also muscle glycogen capacity. Exercise accomplishes both, and as you will learn in Chapter 9, muscle is the metabolic equalizer.

STEP 2: SKIP A MEAL

When you deplete stored glycogen, your body will turn to fat for energy. This produces a by-product called ketones. Your body (including your brain and heart) runs quite well on ketones. In fact, your body was designed to run on ketones whenever glucose levels are low.

> ### KETONES: MISUNDERSTOOD
> # ENERGY.

The problem is that most people never run low on glucose. Every meal contains more than enough starch and sugar to last till the next meal or snack.

So you're saying that producing ketones is a good thing?

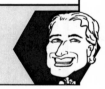

Not only a good thing. Evidence is mounting to show that it is a critical part of high-efficiency metabolism.

Diabetics (especially those with Type 1 diabetes) can sometimes have high levels of ketones in their body. This condition, called ketoacidosis, is a cause for concern because it can indicate that they are ill, have an infection, or that their diabetes is out of control. Thus Type 1 diabetics who have measurable ketones in their blood or urine should speak with their doctor promptly.

This unusual state, however, should not be confused with normal ketosis, which can help us get back in synch with our genes. If our hunting-and-gathering ancestors spent a significant amount of time burning fat and creating ketones, we should at least look to see if this affords some metabolic advantage.

Turns out, it does. A rise in ketone production helps lower blood glucose and insulin. Ketones also raise cellular energy levels while reducing the production of harmful free radicals, meaning that burning fat is highly efficient.[1] What's more, ketones signal the muscles to generate more mitochondria, which are the energy factories within each cell.[2]

Finally, ketones are actually the preferred fuel for the brain. Your brain, after all is a huge consumer of energy. It is only about 2% of your body weight, but uses 20% of the oxygen you inhale and 10% of your glucose stores, just to keep the central nervous system running. Ketones are a more efficient fuel, and this increased efficiency has clear benefits on brain activity, including a reduction in damage and improved repair.[3]

Now, you may have heard that calorie restriction (CR) produces similar metabolic benefits, and it does. But are you prepared to reduce your caloric intake to approximately 900 calories per day in order to achieve these results? The good news is that there is an easier way to burn fat and generate ketones. You don't just skip a meal. It's a mini-fast strategy, and you're sleeping during most of it. We call it KickStart.

The KickStart Strategy

1. Enjoy a high-quality dinner, but avoid dessert and eat nothing after 7:00 p.m. If you experience a gnawing hunger that might interfere with sleep, have protein; some leftover fish from dinner, a small bowl of unsweetened yogurt, or a high-fiber, high-protein snack, aiming for 10 grams of protein and at least 5 grams of fiber.

2. Unless your dinner contained a lot of starch, you are likely to run out of glycogen by 5:00 a.m. Thus by the time you awaken at 6:00 a.m., you will already be in the fasted (fat-burning) state.

3. Have a glass of water.

4. Enjoy a **KickStart Super Shake** (ingredient details in Chapter 8).
   In a shaker bottle, combine:
   - 10-12 oz. water
   - 1 tablespoon (15 mL) MCT oil (Medium Chain Triglycerides)
   - 1 tablespoon liquid L-Carnitine
   - 1 tablespoon powdered maca
   - 1 tablespoon D-Ribose
   - 1 rounded tablespoon of whey-protein isolate, rice, soy, pea or hemp protein
   - 1 tablespoon acacia fiber
   - Optional: 300 mg powdered Cissus quadrangularis

5. Perform some moderate-intensity exercise for 30 to 40 minutes. Brisk walking is fine. This accelerates ketone production, which in turn will suppress your appetite. In fact, you will be surprised at how your desire for food disappears.

6. If you are used to having coffee or tea in the morning, brew yourself a cup, but make it either unsweetened or use a small amount of stevia, xylitol or sucralose.

7. Late morning, you may start feeling hungry. If so, have a green drink; either freshly-juiced greens or one of the powders that are available in health food stores. Just make sure the powdered product has no sweeteners or maltodextrin, is organic, and has a net carb value (Total Carbohydrate minus Dietary Fiber) no more than 2 grams per serving.

8. Have a high-quality lunch at 2:00 p.m.

Congratulations! You just fasted for 19 hours, and you were burning fat for about 9. That will help to maximize energy metabolism in five important ways. You:

1. Reduced caloric intake without the torture of calorie restriction.
2. Burned fat and generated ketones
3. Depleted and restored glycogen to improve metabolic fitness
4. Reduced insulin, glucose and glucose "spikes"
5. Activated mitochondrial biogenesis (the elevated ketones signaled your muscle cells to increase the number and density of energy-producing mitochondria)

KickStart FAQs

#1

Why only a rounded tbsp. of protein in the KickStart Super Shake? Isn't more protein better?

Unless you weigh more than 200 pounds, a rounded tbsp. (yielding 10 to 15g of protein) is all you need. Remember that too much protein can halt ketosis because the liver will convert some of the excess protein to glucose.

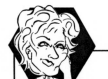

#2

Is the KickStart strategy safe for diabetics?

Diabetics should always check with their physician before making changes in diet and exercise. In my experience, the KickStart strategy can work quite well for those with Type 2 diabetes, especially those who are overweight. Type 2 diabetics should test their blood sugar when they wake up, 20 minutes after exercise, mid-morning and 20 minutes after lunch. You're watching for hypoglycemia (low blood sugar) in the first three readings and a possible elevation in blood sugar after lunch.

#3

What if I'm on a prescribed medication that I take every morning, like thyroid hormones?

Don't ever stop taking a medication prescribed by your physician. If you find that taking your meds on an empty stomach produces discomfort, ask your doctor if you can take them later in the day or take them with the KickStart Super Drink, which contains protein.

#4

How many times/week should I practice KickStart?

We recommend one to three times a week. Many people find that they look forward to their KickStart days because they are more calm (love those ketones) and have better energy and mental clarity. Plus, the Super Shake accelerates muscle gain, strength and stamina, all of which sends positive information to your genome.

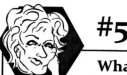

#5

What if I still have carb cravings?

The Metabolic Makeover program generally abolishes carb cravings within a few weeks. But if this continues to be a problem, I recommend:

1. Increasing protein intake.

2. Supplement with 5,000 mcg biotin (available at health food stores) one or two times per day with meals. Biotin is very genoactive, producing multiple metabolic benefits related to glucose balance and the utilization of triglycerides to create energy.[4]

3. Note: most of the time, carb cravings hit late in the day as serotonin levels start to fall. A nutritional supplement known as 5-Hydroxytryptophan or 5-HTP is a precursor to serotonin. 5-HTP also helps with sleep, so the best time to take it is after 5:00 p.m. Start with 100mg, and double that if you're still having trouble walking past that loaf of sourdough bread.

#6

I read that skipping meals causes your body to go into "starvation" mode, preventing weight loss.

That's a common misconception. Because most of us have more than enough glucose and glycogen, you would have to skip a number of meals before there was any adverse effect on metabolism. In addition, the KickStart super shake provides all the protein you need to prevent a "starvation" signal to the genome.

(i)

Summary

1. Human history is filled with periods of scarcity and famine. Thus, we developed effective biochemical strategies for storing energy. Beyond the accumulation of fat, the liver and muscles store glycogen.

2. Hardly anyone today utilizes these survival strategies. In modern industrialized nations, people generally eat more calories than they need, 365 days a year.

3. But what if activating energy storage pathways produced remarkable metabolic benefits? What if this is an essential component of human physiology? Until now, no one was asking these questions.

4. The answer is a resounding YES. We now know that activating energy storage pathways (glycogen and fat-burning):

   A. Improves energy production at the cell level
   B. Reduces inflammation and oxidative stress
   C. Improves insulin sensitivity
   D. Restores glucose balance
   E. Reduces risk for cardiovascular disease
   F. Supports the immune system
   G. Protects beta cells of the pancreas, helping to maintain optimal pancreatic function
   H. Reduces stress on the brain and central nervous system
   I. May reduce risk for neurodegenerative disorders including Alzheimer's and Parkinson's disease [5]

5. Energy storage pathways can be activated by calorie restriction (CR), which is arduous, possibly dangerous and nearly impossible to follow.

6. KickStart is a simple strategy aimed at achieving many of the same benefits, that can be easily be incorporated into one's life.

Endnotes

1 Kim do, Y., Davis, L. M., Sullivan, P. G., Maalouf, M., Simeone, T. A., van-Brederode, J., and Rho, J. M. (2007). Ketone bodies are protective against oxidative stress in neocortical neu- rons. J. Neurochem. 101, 1316–1326.

2 Bough, K. J., Wetherington, J., Has- sel, B., Pare, J. F., Gawryluk, J. W., Greene, J. G., Shaw, R., Smith, Y., Geiger, J. D., and Dingledine, R. J. (2006). Mitochondrial biogenesis in the anticonvulsant mechanism of the ketogenic diet. Ann. Neurol. 60, 223–235.

3 Emily Deans, M.D. http://evolutionarypsychiatry.blogspot.com/2010/08/your-brain-on-ketones.html. Accessed 12/29/12

4 Larrieta E, Velasco F, Vital P, López-Aceves T, Lazo-de-la-Vega-Monroy ML, Rojas A, Fernandez-Mejia C. Pharmacological concentrations of bio- tin reduce serum triglycerides and the expression of lipogenic genes. Eur J Pharmacol. 2010 Oct 10;644(1-3):263-8. doi: 10.1016/j.ejphar.2010.07.009.

5 Henderson ST. Ketone bodies as a therapeutic for Alzheimer's disease. Neurotherapeutics. 2008 Jul;5(3):470-80. doi: 10.1016/j.nurt.2008.05.004. Review. PMID: 18625458

REFLECTIONS

---

1. Assuming you enjoy food security now, how far back in your family tree do you have to go to find the threat of hunger and starvation?

2. Have you tried the eat slow, chew well conscious eating strategy? What did you discover?

3. Why do you think dessert has become such an important part of our eating experience?

Notes:

Chapter Eight

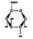

METABOLIC MODIFIERS

We've been dropping hints in previous chapters about natural compounds that can help you eat less, generate more energy, burn fat and increase your strength and stamina. And while that probably sounds familiar, there's one important difference between this chapter and the raft of spam emails you get every day. **This is research, not hype.**

Who did the research?

I am fortunate to be part of an international research group with full-scale genomics, proteomics, biochemical, biological and proton NMR technologies. Add to this an agricultural division with farms in every climate zone, and you have what is probably the most extensive natural products R&D operation in the world.

Natalie is a double board-certified physician who owns one of busiest clinics in the Pacific Northwest specializing in preventive health and anti-aging. We are both info-maniac science nerds, and are constantly reviewing the massive amount of biomedical literature published each month.

We have carefully evaluated the safety and efficacy of each one of these Metabolic Modifiers. The chapter is extensively referenced so that you can discuss these compounds with your doctor or your biochemist brother-in-law. Additionally, we have tested these compounds ourselves. In some cases, it even involved having a 24-hour glucose monitor implanted in my abdomen. Other tests were easier, but in each case, we gained more knowledge regarding Metabolic Modifiers than one could ever get from a medical journal.

The maintenance of high metabolic efficiency requires a multitude of genetic adjustments, including those that promote fat-burning, reduce fat storage, enhance insulin sensitivity and accelerate glucose disposal. Secondary adjustments include those that improve protein synthesis in the liver, uptake by the muscles, and the maintenance of muscle mass with advancing age.

The genes encoding these proteins are in essence the blueprints that we have inherited from our parents.
BUT DNA IS NOT DESTINY.
Each of these genes has a wide functional range, known as gene expression. And gene expression is largely determined by diet and lifestyle.

This chapter is not intended as a recipe for curing diabetes or Metabolic Syndrome. Nor are we suggesting that you consume every one of these compounds in our suggested amount. Instead, this is a catalog of natural product tools for you to consider, based on your needs and with the guidance of a health-care professional.

NOTE: because new research is constantly being published, we recommend you check the Metabolic Modifier section of TheMetabolicMakeover.com for monthly updates.

So with great confidence and joy, we present the compounds that can enable you to do what no previous generation has achieved. The ability to control your metabolism, and experience a higher quality of life than you ever imagined.

The 5 Metabolic Modifiers
THAT IMPROVE CELLULAR ENERGY PRODUCTION

"Well, I just don't have the energy I used to." Doctors hear this complaint more than any other, and until recently, they had no response other than to say (and perhaps you've heard these words yourself) "You're just getting older." Or how about this one: "Learn to live with it."

You see, after ruling out anemia, hypothyroid or a disease-related cause of fatigue, physicians had no solution. And because they themselves were most likely experiencing the same thing, they thought it was pretty much hopeless. All of that changed when scientists—including my research group — discovered nutritional factors that control the efficiency of the Krebs cycle.

The Krebs (or citric acid) cycle is the biochemical assembly line that generates energy within each cell. The energy "factories" where this takes place are called mitochondria (my-toe-KON-dree-ah).

For more than two decades, Bruce Ames and his colleagues at the University of California, Berkeley, looked at the connection between fatigue and mitochondrial efficiency.

They began by comparing the activity levels of young rats vs. old rats. To no one's surprise, they found that young rats were far more active. And here's where the new paradigm of aging comes in. While others made these observations and said, "oh well, that's just the way it is," the Ames group looked for the reason for this decline. In the metabolic model, in other words, there are no assumptions. If aging is associated with increasing fatigue, we should be able to learn the cause. And find a cure.

Breakthrough

Cells make energy through oxidation, a biochemical combustion of the fuel you eat and the oxygen you breathe. The Ames group theorized that over time, the by-products of oxidation might damage the mitochondria, resulting in lower energy production. Think of a factory where the product being produced also causes the machinery to rust. At a certain point, the factory will grind to a halt, and that's exactly what happens to mitochondria. As cellular energy declines, so does organ function. As organ function declines, so does your health. It used to be inevitable, but thanks to Ames and his crew, this critical facet of aging can now be reversed.

1. Acetyl-L-carnitine

In a series of experiments, a team of scientists from five research organizations[1] gave acetyl-L-carnitine and alpha lipoic acid—nutrients found in small amounts in red meat and milk— to older rats. Within seven weeks they saw dramatic improvements in mitochondria function and energy production.[2] This not only led to increased activity levels, but as Dr. Ames stated, "With the two supplements together, these old rats got up and did the macarena. The brain looks better, they are full of energy—everything we looked at looks more like a young animal."[3]

Ames' last point is perhaps the most compelling. Restored energy is important, but to also achieve dramatic improvements in memory was an unexpected and exciting "side-effect." In other words, increasing cellular energy production appears to improve everything.

NOTE: In April 2013, a study was published in Nature Medicine suggesting that carnitine supplementation could increase risk for atherosclerosis.[4] As usual, surprising reports like this need to be viewed in the context of prior research. After looking at all of the facts, Natalie and I conclude that acetyl-L carnitine is safe and beneficial.

In fact, a new meta-analysis of the research on carnitine and heart health was published by researchers from Mayo Clinic. This was a large systematic review of 13 controlled trials that enrolled over 3,600 participants; making it the largest, most powerful scientific review of carnitine's cardiovascular benefits.

The Mayo Clinic study was conducted with people who had experienced a heart attack. In this group, carnitine supplementation was associated with a 27% reduction in all-cause mortality, a 65% reduction in ventricular arrhythmias, and a 40% reduction in chest pain symptoms.

These impressive benefits occurred via increased mitochondrial energy production and improved circulation. The authors describe carnitine as an inexpensive therapy with an "excellent safety profile."[5]

Suggested use: 500-1,000mg/day. A must for vegetarians and others who don't eat red meat.

---

2. Alpha Lipoic Acid (ALA)

Alpha lipoic acid is a vitamin-like compound produced within mitochondria, where it acts as a regulating coenzyme. A form of alpha lipoic acid is found in foods like brewer's yeast, liver, kidney, spinach, broccoli and potatoes, but none of the food sources actually raise tissue levels of ALA. Thus, virtually all alpha lipoic acid available today is created in a laboratory.

ALA is a spectacular antioxidant. While some antioxidants like vitamin C work only in water, and others like vitamin E work only in fatty tissues, ALA is both water and fat soluble, meaning that it can work throughout the body. What's more, it can rejuvenate other antioxidants and potentiates the benefits of alpha ketoglutaric acid (AKG).[6]

And that's just for starters. Alpha lipoic acid enhances energy production by stimulating AMPK, and as you would guess, also improves glucose disposal, making it a remarkably effective nutrient for anyone with prediabetes, type 2 diabetes or Metabolic Syndrome.

If that's not enough reason to supplement with alpha lipoic acid, it can also help you lose weight by telling the liver and muscles to burn fat. And remember the biodialog in Chapter Four, where adipose cells were off-loading fat into adjacent muscle, causing damage and destruction? Alpha lipoic acid prevents that.[7] Research has also revealed ALA benefits in immunity, strength, endurance and cardiovascular health.[8]

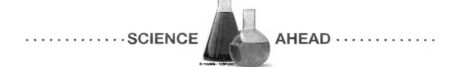

· · · · · · · · · · · · SCIENCE   AHEAD · · · · · · · · · · · ·

"Lipoic acid supplementation improved body composition, glucose tolerance, and energy expenditure. Lipoic acid increased skeletal muscle mitochondrial biogenesis with increased phosphorylation of AMPK and messenger RNA expression of PGC-1alpha and glucose transporter-4."

WANG Y, LI X, GUO Y, CHAN L, GUAN X. ALPHA-LIPOIC ACID INCREASES ENERGY EXPENDITURE BY ENHANCING AMPK-PEROXI-SOME PROLIFERATOR-ACTIVATED RECEPTOR-GAMMA COACTIVATOR-1ALPHA SIGNALING IN THE SKELETAL MUSCLE OF AGED MICE. METABOLISM. 2010 JUL;59(7):967-76.

Translation: Alpha lipoic acid has been shown in animals and humans to be a potent and multi-faceted Metabolic Modifier.

NOTE: for alpha lipoic acid aficionados: a more potent form of ALA is showing up in health food stores, called R+alpha lipoic acid or r-ALA. This appears to be nearly 100% bioactive, whereas standard ALA is about 60% bioactive. Since the r-ALA is more than double the cost of standard ALA however, Natalie and I continue to use standard ALA. Importantly, more than 90% of the published human research on alpha lipoic acid has used standard ALA. Now, when someone tries to sell you r-ALA, claiming that it is the only bioactive form, you can make an informed choice.

> **Suggested use:** 100mg to 500mg of alpha lipoic acid per day best taken in divided doses. If using r-lipoic acid, you can use less.

3. Alpha-Ketoglutaric Acid

Although it sounds like something from a chemist's lab, alpha-Ketoglutaric acid (AKG) is an essential nutrient found in every cell of the human body. In fact, AKG is the rate-limiting step in the Krebs cycle, meaning that an insufficient level can dramatically reduce cellular energy production. The best news? You can eat it. Human clinical trials have documented improvements in exercise ability and recovery time with AKG supplementation.[9,10]

> *"This study has shown that nutritional supplementation with α-keto acids in healthy, untrained subjects significantly improved exercise tolerance, training effects, and [post-exercise] recovery."*
>
> LIU Y, LANGE R, ET AL. IMPROVED TRAINING TOLERANCE BY SUPPLEMENTATION WITH A-KETO ACIDS IN UNTRAINED YOUNG ADULTS: A RANDOMIZED, DOUBLE BLIND, PLACEBO-CONTROLLED TRIAL. J INT SOC SPORTS NUTR. 2012 AUG 2;9(1):37. DOI: 10.1186/1550-2783-9-37.

Suggested use: Natalie recommends 200 to 500mg per day for general energy support, and to double that on strenuous exercise days.

---

4. D-Ribose

Every "turn" of the Krebs cycle produces an energy molecule known as ATP (adenosine tri-phosphate). At the split second that three phosphate ions are released, they are fused together with adenosine and ribose. Viola ATP! Couch potatoes rarely lack ribose but anyone who is strenuously active usually needs more. Thus, providing a ready pool of ribose allows you to optimize ATP production.[11] D-Ribose can also help during periods of intense stress.[12]

Suggested use: I use 1 to 6g per day of D-Ribose with sports/fitness professionals. Natalie recommends up to 5g per day for her patients with heart disease.[13]

---

5. Medium Chain Triglycerides (a.k.a. MCTs)

Dietary fats and oils are made of triglycerides, structures that contain three fatty acids attached to one glycerol molecule. Tri-glyceride, get it? These form chains containing 4 to 26 carbon atoms, with hydrogen atoms attached to them. The reason for this mini lipid lesson is that fats are classified according to the number of carbon atoms they contain. You will hear about short chain triglycerides (fewer than 6 carbons), medium chain triglycerides (6 to 12 carbons) and long chain triglycerides (ranging from 12 to 26 carbons). The vast majority of the fats and oils you eat, whether from an animal or a plant, are long-chain triglycerides.

What is special about MCTs (derived from coconut and palm kernel oil) is that they are easier to digest, absorb rapidly into the bloodstream, and are used primarily to provide energy rather than adding to your waistline. In fact, studies show that consuming MCTs can help you lose weight.[14,15] That happens because they increase fat burning and exercise tolerance.[16]

Because of this energy factor, MCTs are used by lots of people. Physicians use purified MCTs to help nourish premature infants. If you were recovering from a serious injury or infection, you most likely would be given MCTs in the Intensive Care Unit. Athletes use MCTs to increase stamina, and this remarkable Metabolic Modifier is turning out to be a key feature in *The Metabolic Makeover*.

> **Suggested use:** MCT oil is available in health food stores, and because of its neutral taste, can be added to a smoothie, shake, or mixed with your salad dressing. We include a tbsp. in our KickStart Super-Shake (see Chapter Seven).

The 3 Metabolic Modifiers
That Increase Fat Burning

A naturally thin person and an overweight friend enter a restaurant. They both weigh the same (in terms of pounds). They order the same meal and eat the same number of calories. The naturally-thin person leaves the restaurant a little warmer. The other leaves the restaurant a little fatter.

The process of producing cellular energy in the form of heat is called thermogenesis. If you didn't inherit the ability to easily and rapidly convert calories to heat, there are Metabolic Modifiers that can help you do just that.

Green tea and bitter orange (citrus aurantium) stimulate thermogenesis via the central nervous system. Used in moderation, they can be very effective, as they do not cause the rapid heart beat and elevated blood pressure like CNS stimulant drugs and now-banned ephedra supplements.

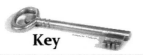
Key

Calories do matter, but clearly, what is more important is the fate of those calories. When naturally-thin people consume a meal, there are "energy sensors" with biochemical names like AMPK and adiponectin which determine how much to use and how much to store. If you didn't win the DNA Lottery, and have low levels of these energy sensors, you will tend to store calories instead of burning them.

But, as we've shared, DNA is not destiny. A number of Metabolic Modifiers work by stimulating AMPK or raising levels of adiponectin. A primary example of this is:

1. Fucoxanthin (derived from brown seaweed)

Research shows that by stimulating AMPK, fucoxanthin can help people lose weight and also maintain ideal weight.[17] Importantly, fucoxanthin works directly in fat cells. By targeting energy distribution at the mitochondrial level, this non-stimulating activity provides an important new tool to achieve successful long-term weight management.

> **Suggested use:** And you don't need much. Effective products available today include anywhere from 5 to 15mg per day.

2. Green (Unroasted) Coffee Bean

This is another Metabolic Modifier that raises AMPK. This occurs via a compound known as chlorogenic acid, found in green coffee bean but destroyed during roasting.[18] In true Metabolic Makeover fashion, chlorogenic acid has also been shown to improve glucose balance and exercise tolerance.[19]

> **Suggested use:** 100 to 500mg per day

We've talked a lot about how natural products can activate metabolic signals in tissues throughout the body. These signaling molecules can be genes (like ANGPTL4), hormones (like adiponectin) or an enzyme like AMPK.

3. Omega-3 Fatty acids from fish oil, krill or algae

These have been shown to stimulate all three of the above pathways, producing benefits for people who want to lose weight, build muscle, and reduce their risk for cardiovascular disease at the same time.[20,21] The most important omega-3 fatty acids are EPA and DHA.

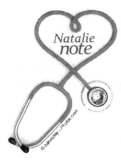

My patients are often surprised by my advice to supplement with fat (fish oil) in order to lose weight. But EPA and DHA are an essential component of any comprehensive fat-loss program. Suggested use: 1 to 4g per day.

Is there a fish-oil "controversy?" Not really.

In 2012, a study published in the Journal of the American Medical Association, concluded that supplementing with omega-3 fatty acids (a.k.a. fish oil), is not associated with a reduction in risk for major cardiovascular events.[22]

Headlines appeared, written by journalists (who didn't read or understand the study) announcing, "Fish oil doesn't work."

Those who read and understood the study would certainly disagree. Here's why. The study was a statistical analysis combining the results from 20 previous clinical trials. This is called a meta-analysis. They looked for the incidence of cardiovascular events (all-cause mortality, cardiac death, sudden death, heart attack and stroke) in people taking omega-3 fatty acids vs. people not taking these supplements.

Importantly, the vast majority of these studies were secondary prevention trials, meaning the subjects had pre-existing cardiovascular disease. That also means that virtually every subject was already on a number of drugs, including a statin, aspirin, a blood thinner and one or more drugs to control blood pressure. What's more, the amount of omega-3 fatty acids used by these subjects varied widely—from 1 to 4g per day.

> **Suggested use:** reading hundreds of prior studies that strongly support the cardiovascular benefits of omega-3 fatty acids, Natalie and I conclude that:
>
> 1. The effective dose is 3 to 5g, depending on how many servings of fish a person consumes, per week.
>
> 2. Omega-3 fatty acids are probably more effective as primary prevention; that is taken before you have cardiovascular disease.

The 8 Metabolic Modifiers
THAT IMPROVE GLUCOSE METABOLISM

NOTE: These natural products have been shown to reduce blood sugar and insulin. If you are under the care of a physician for diabetes or hypoglycemia, you must consult with your doctor before using these Metabolic Modifiers. The good news is that none of them produce rapid or drastic effects. They work by improving energy metabolism, which is a gradual process.

1. Aloe

There is no longer any doubt that aloe is a true Metabolic Modifier. In a placebo-controlled human clinical trial with 72 diabetic patients, the treatment group consumed 15 milliliters (a little over 3 teaspoons) of aloe gel twice per day. After 42 days, blood sugar in the treatment group was reduced 43 percent and triglycerides were reduced by 44 percent.[23]

In people with prediabetes, consuming an aloe vera complex for 8 weeks produced remarkable metabolic improvements, including reduced LDL, fasting glucose, insulin, HgbA1C and markers of oxidative stress.[24] Follow-up research (also a placebo-controlled human clinical trial) not only confirmed these metabolic benefits, but documented reduced body fat and increased muscle mass in the treatment group consuming an aloe complex compared to controls.[25]

There are a variety of aloe products on the market today. Best are those certified for purity and potency by the International Aloe Science Council (IASC).

Suggested use: 2 to 6 oz. of aloe-vera juice per day or the equivalent in dried concentrate capsules.

---

2. Chromium

Chromium's metabolic importance stems primarily from the co-factor role it plays with insulin. Since insulin is required for the delivery of fuel to brain and muscles, insufficient chromium can contribute to fatigue and low metabolic efficiency. Research conducted by the US Department of Agriculture found that 90% of the people studied were obtaining inadequate levels of chromium from their diet.[26] Diabetics usually have low levels of chromium compared to people without that disease.[27] Importantly, supplementation has been shown to correct chromium deficiency and improve insulin sensitivity.[28]

There's a lot of hype flying around in the popular press, and this has created confusion as to the best form of chromium to use. Some manufacturers simply list "chromium" on their label, leaving in doubt the true bioavailability and safety of the product. Others list "GTF chromium," while still others use the term "trivalent chromium," which simply differentiates it from the industrial chromium that coats the bumper of your car.

One excellent research-proven, biologically-active compound is Chromium polynicotinate; that is, chromium bound to the essential vitamin, niacin. This compound is consistent with the highest standards of purity, potency and effectiveness. "Nicotinate" refers to niacin (vitamin B-3) not nicotine.

> **Suggested use:** 50 to 200 mcg per day.

3. Vanadium

This is another trace mineral with the ability to improve insulin sensitivity. Recent research shows that it works independently of chromium but the best results can be achieved when used together.[29]

> **Suggested use:** 50 to 200 mcg per day.

"One out of every five Americans has metabolic syndrome. It affects 40% of people in their 60s and 70s. Insulin resistance, with or without the presence of metabolic syndrome, significantly increases the risk of cardiovascular disease."

A SCIENTIFIC REVIEW: THE ROLE OF CHROMIUM
IN INSULIN RESISTANCE. DIABETES EDUC. 2004;
SUPPL:2-14.

4. Banaba (Lagerstroemia speciosa)

Banaba is an herb that supports metabolic fitness in two ways: Human clinical trials show that it helps to normalize blood sugar[30] and cell culture analysis demonstrates that it can inhibit the formation of new fat cells. Because of these benefits, a study in the *Journal of Nutrition* concluded that "Banaba may be useful for prevention and treatment of hyperglycemia and obesity in type 2 diabetics."[31]

> **Suggested use:** Natalie recommends a leaf extract standardized for corosolic acid at 50 to 200 mg per day.

5. Berberine

It's been said that nature color-codes medicinal plants, and that is certainly true of Berberine, a bright yellow compound found in the Berberis family of plants, including Berberis aquifolium (Oregon grape), Berberis vulgaris (barberry), and Berberis aristata (tree turmeric). Berberine also gives the medicinal herb golden seal its golden color, and lends its hue to the petals of the California poppy.

Traditionally, Berberine has been used for its anti-fungal and anti-microbial activity, but researchers are now focusing on its ability to improve insulin sensitivity and blood-sugar balance. In human clinical trials, Berberine was effective when used alone, when combined with lifestyle modification, and when combined with diabetes drugs such as Metformin.[32]

New research shows that Berberine is very genoactive. It stimulates AMPK in liver and muscle, increases expression of genes involved in fat burning, and down-regulates genes involved in fat storage. It doesn't get much better than that.[33]

> **Suggested use:** Natalie recommends 200 to 500 mg 20 minutes before meals for her patients with blood-sugar issues.

6. GABA

Gamma aminobutyric acid (GABA) is a non protein-forming amino acid that acts as a neurotransmitter in the brain. It is generally considered to have an inhibitory function, producing a calming effect. When GABA receptors were found in the gut as well as the brain, researchers started to look for additional effects. In animal experiments, an oral dose of GABA produces profound metabolic benefits including: reduced inflammation, improved insulin sensitivity, normalization of blood sugar and a reduction of fat storage. As a result, mice fed a high-fat diet supplemented with GABA simply do not gain weight.[34]

> **Suggested use:** Natalie recommends 200 to 500 mg per day for her patients with poor glucose metabolism; double that for those with stress or anxiety eating behavior.

7. Panax (red Korean) ginseng

Panax ginseng is probably the most misunderstood Metabolic Modifier because of the hype surrounding this ancient root. In the 70s, everyone thought it was an aphrodisiac (for men only, because of the shape of the root). In the 80s, research started to confirm true energy benefits, but people assumed Panax was a stimulant. That myth persists to this day, only because it is often combined with "energy" drinks and products that contain caffeine and other stimulants.

Fact is, Panax ginseng doesn't increase cortisol levels—as botanical and drug stimulants do—and has actually been shown to lower blood pressure and heart rate in human clinical trials.[35]

So what makes Panax ginseng a Metabolic Modifier?

1. Clear anti-fatigue benefits have been found in a placebo-controlled human clinical trial. Researchers documented performance improvements in physical and mental tasks.[36]

2. Panax ginseng can also improve glucose metabolism via improvements in insulin sensitivity.[37]

3. Panax ginseng stimulates production of AMPK, thus providing a third bioenergetic mode of action that enhances exercise tolerance.[38]

4. Panax ginseng is an amazing antioxidant that protects cells and their mitochondria. At the same time, Panax restores the activity of other antioxidant enzymes.[39] In animal experiments, these antioxidant effects have been shown to protect the brain from altered blood flow and oxygen delivery associated with aging.[40]

5. Panax has been a treatment for type 2 diabetes for centuries, and we now know that it effectively protects pancreatic beta cells under high-glucose conditions.[41]

6. And yes, while it may not be an aphrodisiac, Panax ginseng has been shown to be an effective treatment for erectile dysfunction in placebo-controlled human clinical trials.[42,43]

NOTE ON PURITY AND POTENCY: The value of ginseng roots increases with the age of the plant, with the highest concentration of active compounds (known as ginsenosides) appearing after year three. Many experts believe that seven-year-old roots are the most valuable. But ginseng (especially when grown as a monocrop) is susceptible to a variety of fungal infections. So imagine the dilemma for the grower, needing to protect plants for 3 to 7 years, during which time the entire crop can be destroyed by any number of fungi that attack the root or leaves.

Thus it is common for growers throughout the world to use fungicides on the growing crop. In the best case, growers apply the appropriate amount at the appropriate time, at least a month before harvest. But in 1998, lab tests revealed widespread contamination of imported ginseng. It was learned that Quintozene (pentachloronitrobenzene) was being applied to the plants right before harvest, and even applied to the harvested root.[44]

Today, major national brands all test for chemical residue. So that takes care of the purity issue. What about potency? Natalie and I strongly suggest, not only looking for a leading national brand, but a product standardized for a specific concentration of ginsenosides. When in doubt, look for this information on the company's website or contact them directly.

Suggested use: Look for a minimum of 3% ginsenosides. At this concentration, capsules containing 200 to 600 mg are available. Leading suppliers also offer a variety of concentrates, ranging from 3 to 1 (labeled 3:1) to 5:1. At these higher potency concentrations, capsules containing 100 to 300 mg are available. Follow label instructions for suggested use.

Some people prefer to chew on the actual root, available dried or sliced and flavored. Follow the same guidelines regarding purity and potency (e.g., does the manufacturer test for chemical residue, and how old are the roots?).

8. Berries and cherries

In addition to berberine's bright yellow pigments, Metabolic Modifiers are also found in deep purple and blue fruits and vegetables. A study published in the *Journal of Nutrition* found that participants who drank two blueberry shakes daily for six weeks experienced a significant improvement in insulin sensitivity.[45]

Further research has identified the specific compounds from blueberry responsible for this remarkable benefit. Anthocyanins (also found in other purple and blue fruits, as well as cranberry, black cherry and eggplant peel) were associated with a reduced risk for type 2 diabetes in a massive diet analysis of more than 200,000 men and women.[46]

> **Suggested use:** Include deep blue and red fruits and vegetables in your daily diet and/or supplement with concentrates that retain these valuable anthocyanins.

The 12 Metabolic Modifiers
THAT SUPPORT EXERCISE AND MUSCLE MASS

1. I love Leucine

In *The Metabolic Plan* (Ballantine 2003) I touted the muscle support benefits of Branched Chain Amino Acids (BCAAs). Of the three BCAA's (leucine, isoleucine and valine), only leucine has the capacity to directly stimulate muscle protein synthesis (MPS).[47] In animal studies, leucine has also been found to slow the degeneration of muscle tissue that occurs in the aging process.[48] So, since it appears that leucine provides 90% of the metabolic benefits delivered by the BCAAs, it only makes sense to maximize efficiency with a leucine supplement. The good news is that, since leucine comprises only 5 to 10% of dietary protein, even small amounts of additional leucine can make a difference.

Natalie note I've been asked why I recommend a leucine supplement instead of the addition of whole protein. The answer is twofold. First, you get more muscle-protein-synthesis bang for your buck with leucine, and more important, animal studies demonstrate that eating grain and bean proteins fail to increase MPS. Only egg and whey sources of leucine stimulated MPS in a recent study published in *Nutrition and Metabolism*.[49]

Suggested use: 500 to 1,000 mg per day. Vegans may need more, especially after age 40.

---

2. Creatine

In the late 1920s, researchers were puzzled by the fact that they could exercise lab rats to complete exhaustion, but even when the rats could no longer move, their heart and chest muscles continued to pump oxygen and fuel. What was it about these muscles that allowed them to continue functioning when all their adenosine tri-phosphate (ATP) had been depleted? This led to the discovery of an energy reserve called phosphocreatine.

Turns out that under conditions of strenuous exertion, phosphocreatine donates a phosphate ion to ADP (adenosine diphosphate) thus creating more ATP (adenosine triphosphate). It was not until the 1992 Olympics in Barcelona however, that people learned that some athletes were taking creatine and achieving impressive gains in strength and stamina. A year later, the first creatine supplements appeared on health-food store shelves. As you can guess, I've been following the science and the hype around creatine very carefully. We now know a great deal about the compound, and there is some new information that you probably have not heard.

Is creatine only for bodybuilders?

We are all bodybuilders. Every adult replaces about 300 billion cells a day. We are all, in other words, building a new body. The problem is that building and maintaining muscle becomes more difficult the older we get. So I consider creatine to be an anti-aging ingredient that also helps athletes, bodybuilders, and your average aging Joe/Jane.

NOTE: Do I need to point out that creatine won't do anything for you if you sit on the couch? It will not move your thumbs more rapidly over the controller of a video game, nor allow you to surf more Internet sites. Creatine—and in fact, all Metabolic Modifiers—work only when you work. The good news is that with adequate creatine, you are far more likely to get results (measurable increase in muscle strength and definition), and that is powerfully motivating.

Is there anything that will maximize the benefits of creatine supplementation?

Yes. Research shows that better results can be obtained by taking alpha lipoic acid (100 to 500 mg) at the same time.[50]

> **Suggested use:** When starting creatine supplementation, research suggests a larger dose (5g twice per day) for the first 5 to 7 days, produces better results. After that, a single 5g dose will maintain the increased muscle power.

3. Beta Alanine

Beta alanine, a modified form of the amino acid alanine, has been touted by bodybuilders as the next big thing (after creatine). But like creatine, it's perhaps more valuable for anti-aging. Here's why.

Remember in Chapter 5 our discussion of the damaging process known as glycation? Oh, you didn't read Chapter 5...skipped right to Metabolic Modifiers? O.K. to review: when blood sugar is elevated, the sugar (glucose and especially fructose) starts reacting with (think: altering/inactivating) proteins. The most well-known of these altered proteins is glycosylated hemoglobin, otherwise known as hemoglobin A1c or simply HbA1c.

But glycation is not just a problem for diabetics who have hemoglobin that can no longer ferry oxygen to their cells. It's a problem for everyone as we age. Advanced Glycation Endproducts (aptly abbreviated AGEs) contribute to atherosclerosis, cardiovascular disease, cancer, and obviously, diabetes.

In Chapter 5, we advised you to reduce glycation by avoiding refined sugars and high-heat cooking. Here's another tip: carnosine, a nutrient found primarily in meat, fish and dairy foods, can prevent glycation. In fact, it also protects blood vessels and the heart, increases stamina and endurance, protects the brain and acts as a powerful antioxidant.[51,52,53]

A little detail (deep breath)....

Carnosine is a dipeptide, meaning that it is composed of two amino acids, beta alanine and histidine. Beta alanine is the rate-limiting component, meaning that carnosine synthesis is limited by the amount of available beta alanine. Thus supplementing with beta alanine is actually a better strategy than taking carnosine pills.[54,55] Beta alanine will increase the concentration of carnosine in your muscles, resulting in greater strength and endurance.[56,57] More important for those of us not trying out for the Olympics, it will make exercise feel easier, delay aging, and may even help prevent Alzheimer's.

NOTE: Your muscles love beta alanine, and supplemental beta alanine tends to be taken up rather quickly by the muscles. Early on, Natalie and I noticed that any excess that remained in the bloodstream would cause a prickly feeling on the skin; a condition called paresthesia. Since it is harmless and abates in less than an hour, we now use this phenomenon as a cheap and fast test for muscle mass and muscle quality.

For example, I weigh 170 pounds and have a relatively high muscle-to-fat ratio. More important, my insulin sensitivity is high. Another way to say that is: I have low insulin resistance, meaning that my muscles have no problem taking up amino acids like beta alanine. Thus I can take a whopping 2.5-gram (2,500 mg) dose of beta alanine and feel nothing.

Natalie weighs 150 and still has some insulin resistance. When she takes 1.5 grams (1,500 mg) her skin feels prickly and her face feels hot for about an hour. Fortunately, this doesn't happen when she takes 750 mg.

You can even do this beta-alanine "test" yourself to evaluate your muscle mass, muscle quality and insulin status. A woman weighing 140 pounds who experiences a transient paresthesia with 500 mg of beta alanine is very likely to have insufficient muscle mass and/or insulin-resistant muscle cells. Your beta-alanine "tolerance" will improve as you increase muscle mass and take some Metabolic Modifiers like chromium, vanadium, alpha lipoic acid and Banaba.

> **Suggested use:** women should generally start with a single dose of 500 mg of beta alanine. This can be repeated two or even three times per day for optimal results. Men can usually start with 750 to 1500 mg two to three times per day. Doses should be at least two hours apart to avoid paresthesia.

4. Cissus quadrangularis

Cissus quadrangularis (CQ) is an herb native to Africa and Southeast Asia. It has a thousand-year history in ancient medical traditions, and was used primarily to strengthen bones and accelerate the healing of fractures. In the last decade, researchers have confirmed that benefit, and intrigued by this anabolic (build and repair) activity, looked for a mode of action. Turns out CQ stimulates repair at the DNA level, and would be expected to strengthen other connective tissue including tendons, ligaments and muscles.[58] This is important for anyone involved in strenuous resistance exercise with machines or free weights.

Another benefit has recently been discovered for CQ. Placebo-controlled human trials found that cissus is a reliable and safe weight-loss aid.[59] The mode of action? Improving insulin sensitivity and decreasing appetite. [60,61]

> **Suggested use:** 200 to 300 mg per day.

5. HMB (Hydroxy Methylbutyrate)

You are probably aware that most advances in metabolic nutrition come from two sources (where people have an intense interest in human performance): the military and sports competition. I've been involved in this arena long enough to have seen scores of compounds discovered, developed, tested, used, and often banned either for adverse side effects or because they produce an unfair drug-induced advantage for the user. The 2013 USADA banned list contains over a hundred anabolic steroids, hormones, growth factors, stimulants, and pharmaceutical drugs.

HMB has not been banned and is widely available in health-food stores, even though it has been shown to enhance strength, stamina and muscle mass.[62], It's not banned because it's a metabolite of leucine, my favorite amino acid (see "I Love Leucine", above).

Best of all, HMB has been shown to be of value for non-athletes, and appears to be one of the best Metabolic Modifiers for men and women over 50. That's because in addition to its anabolic (build, repair) activity, HMB also reduces catabolic damage.[63,64] We must remember that to tip the damage/repair seesaw in our favor, it is best to improve both sides.

> **Suggested use:** 2 to 3 g of HMB per day, in divided doses with food.

6. Maca

Maca is a South American herb with more legend than science. Still, Natalie and I are inquisitive, especially since the folklore revolves around libido and sexual function. Below is the translation of a recent study on Maca, published in Dutch. And, as is often the case, when you ask Google to translate a foreign document, the results can be hilarious. Enjoy.

> *Title: Maca makes cyclists faster and wellustiger*
> *Abstract: "If trained cyclists or triathletes two weeks consecutive maca swallow - Scientific name:Lepidium meyenii , they are not only faster but they also get more sex."*
>
> *J ETHNOPHARMACOL. 2009 SEPTEMBER 22.*

As it turns out, the cyclists did experience greater endurance, but the researchers in that study only measured libido or sexual desire. A few months later the study was published in English.[65]

This is not the only study to show the value of Maca supplements. Animal studies demonstrate that the endurance and energy benefits derive from Maca's antioxidant activity and improved glucose metabolism.[66,67]

Good news is that Maca is widely available as whole powdered root, as well as a variety of concentrates.

> **Suggested use:** Natalie and I use a comprehensive energy stick that contains 750 mg of a potent 4:1 extract, and on weekends, add a spoonful of standard powder to our morning KickStart Super-Shake.

7. Rhodiola

Rhodiola is another exotic root extract with a long history of use for improvements in mood, stamina and energy. Like Maca, there is a growing body of science to support the folklore.

* One mechanism of action (MOA) appears to be an improvement in glucose metabolism in muscle cells, leading to improved ATP production. This is accomplished by up-regulating our good friend, the much-appreciated enzyme known as AMPK.[68]

* Rhodiola also acts as an adaptogen, with human clinical trials showing not only improved stamina, but reduced perception of effort. This is a critical benefit for anyone starting an exercise program.[69]

* Rhodiola also has something to offer elite athletes; faster recovery and reduced muscle damage after strenuous training.[70,71]

Suggested use: Like Maca, rhodiola is available as powdered dried root and in a variety of standardized extracts and concentrates. I recommend 200 to 500 mg per day of rhodiola powder, and up to a gram (1,000 mg) per day for men and women starting an exercise program or engaged in strenuous fitness training.

---

8. Magnesium

Surveys show that half of American adults consume less than the recommended amount of this important mineral. This makes optimal energy production impossible, since magnesium is required for both aerobic and anaerobic energy production. Even slight deficiencies of magnesium have been shown to reduce exercise tolerance.[72]

"Low magnesium intakes and blood levels have been associated with type 2 diabetes, metabolic syndrome, elevated C-reactive protein, hypertension, athero-sclerotic vascular disease, sudden cardiac death, osteoporosis, migraine headache, asthma, and colon cancer."

ROSANOFF A, WEAVER CM, RUDE RK. SUBOPTIMAL MAGNESIUM STATUS IN THE UNITED STATES: ARE THE HEALTH CONSEQUENCES UNDERESTIMATED? NUTR REV. 2012 MAR;70(3):153-64.

Suggested use: Natalie recommends a highly varied natural foods diet that includes magnesium-rich foods like almonds, peanut butter, sunflower seeds, buckwheat, kale and spinach. In addition, she suggests supplementing with 200 to 500 mg of magnesium, and notes that 500 mg at bedtime can improve sleep quality.

---

9. L-Arginine with a special note on weight loss

Maca, rhodiola, HMB, beta alanine and cissus can foster exercise-induced muscle gains. But people on weight-loss diets usually lose a significant amount of muscle no matter how much they exercise. Extra protein can help reduce this loss, but new research demonstrates that supplemental arginine can literally halt muscle loss altogether.

In a placebo-controlled study reported in the journal Amino Acids, researchers put a group of obese men on a weight-loss diet with 45 minutes of exercise twice a day. As you'd expect, everyone lost weight, but men in the arginine group lost more weight than those in the placebo group. More important, men in the placebo group lost more than 3.5 pounds of muscle, which was 43% of their total

weight loss. **A r g h !** Men supplementing with arginine lost...
d r u m   r o l l ... NO muscle. Every ounce they
lost came from fat.[73]

More on Arginine

Natalie and I have debated how much genomic information to
include in this book, since it is rather technical. Hopefully, you
have found it intriguing. Nutrigenomics is now an exploding
area of research around the world as we learn how food affects
signaling molecules that control cell, organ, and tissue function.

We've mentioned about a dozen key genes or signaling molecules that have a profound effect on metabolism. These include:

- NOS: plays a key metabolic role in muscle, heart, blood
  vessels and adipose tissue
- PGC-1alpha: regulates production of mitochondria (the
  energy factories within your cells)
- NRF-2: activates antioxidant enzymes
- PPAR alpha: regulates the transport and utilization of fat
  to create energy
- UCP-1: plays a critical role in thermogenesis; converting
  calories to heat instead of fat
- AMPK: key energy sensor facilitating the use of fat to create energy instead of storage in adipose tissue

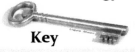
Key

L-Arginine favorably affects the expression and activity of each
of these.[74]

> **Suggested use:** 1 to 3 g per day. If you are on a
> weight loss diet, 2-4 g per day.

10. CoQ10

This essential nutrient is needed for cellular respiration. Every cell of your body—from the top of your head to the tips of your toes—breathes. Energy is produced when oxygen is combined with fuel derived from food and this biochemical "combustion" is sparked by Coenzyme Q10 (CoQ10).

CoQ10 is normally obtained from a group of nutrients known as ubiquinones, which are reduced or destroyed in a highly-processed diet. What's more, CoQ10 levels tend to decrease rapidly with age. 65-year-olds have only about 20% of the CoQ10 they had in their prime.[75]

> **Suggested use:** 30 to 100 mg per day for healthy men and women up to age 50. For those over 50, 200 mg per day. And for people with any type of heart condition: 300 to 400 mg per day.

Natalie note New research is showing that Vitamin D3 may be a Metabolic Modifier. In addition to its myriad benefits throughout the body, Vitamin D3 appears to reduce muscle damage resulting from strenuous exercise.[76] Because Stephen and I promote High Intensity Interval Training (HIIT) (see Chapter 9), this new research underscores my recommendation to include serum Vitamin D in your annual physical exam/blood test. Research suggests that the optimum range is 50 to 80 ng/mL. To maintain that optimum blood level, some people have to supplement with 2,000 to as much as 5,000 iu per day of vitamin D3.

11. DHEA – The King of Metabolic Modifiers

Those familiar with my previous books no doubt understand my obsession with this pro-hormone. It is, after all, the most comprehensive and powerful repair signal in the human body and brain. You also know that DHEA levels fall after age 30 and that the decline becomes steeper with every decade of life, until at age 75, most people are producing only 10 to 20% of the DHEA they produced in their 20s.[77] There is no biochemical in the human body that declines as rapidly, nor one whose decline can have such catastrophic consequences. Restoring DHEA is like amplifying the body's energy and vitality machinery, and it can be done safely.

In The DHEA Breakthrough (Ballantine, 1996), I proposed that this decline is actually a causative factor in declining metabolic fitness, and not simply an effect of the aging process. In *The Metabolic Plan* (Ballantine, 2003) I provided a mountain of evidence to support that position.

We know that people with metabolic syndrome have lower levels of DHEA compared to people the same age without that condition.[78] We know that obese women have lower levels of DHEA compared to lean women of the same age. And we have seen that supplementing with DHEA can improve insulin sensitivity, protein synthesis, muscle mass, bone density and exercise tolerance.[79,80,81]

> *"A major challenge in preventing an epidemic of [muscle loss]-induced frailty in the future is developing public health interventions that deliver an anabolic stimulus to the muscle of elderly adults on a mass scale."*
>
> ROUBENOFF R. SARCOPENIA: A MAJOR MODIFIABLE CAUSE OF FRAILTY IN THE ELDERLY. J NUTR HEALTH AGING 2000;4(3):140-2

Human clinical trials have also shown that DHEA supplements reduce inflammation[82] and even improve exercise tolerance in patients with chronic obstructive pulmonary disease (COPD).[83] Elderly women engaged in an exercise program did poorly if their DHEA blood levels were low. Those with higher levels of DHEA saw improvements in insulin sensitivity, cholesterol, blood pressure, reaction time and stamina.[84]

Researchers at the National Institute of Mental Health even used DHEA to treat what they termed midlife dysthymia, otherwise known as the "blahs." They conclude:

> "A robust effect of DHEA on mood was observed. . . . The symptoms that improved most significantly were anhedonia [lack of pleasure], loss of energy, lack of motivation, emotional "numbness," sadness, inability to cope, and worry."[85]

There is not enough room in this book to detail the myriad ways that DHEA supports and maintains high metabolic efficiency. Since The DHEA Breakthrough, more than 7,000 studies have been published exploring the effect of DHEA on virtually every aspect of energy production, storage, and utilization. As it turns out, DHEA has a synergistic relationship with a number of Metabolic Modifiers.

In section I, we discussed the benefits of acetyl-L-carnitine. New research shows that declining DHEA levels are associated with a subsequent decline in carnitine-driven fat burning.[86] Restoring optimal DHEA levels can have a profound effect on energy and weight management. Remember that fat burning produces energy but also requires energy to get started. Thus, the accumulation of fat with advancing age is a vicious cycle involving low DHEA, reduced energy production, and a sedentary lifestyle. To simply blame weight gain on the lifestyle or the number of calories consumed is unfair and unscientific because it ignores the underlying metabolic defect produced by low levels of DHEA.

So, does taking DHEA correct this defect and support weight loss?

In the International Journal of Obesity, we read: "Regarding the action of DHEA as a fat-reducing hormone, it is possible that this hormone reduces the peripheral requirement for insulin by increasing glucose disposal, and that lower insulin levels are associated with a higher plasma ratio between lipolytic hormones and insulin, and a higher efficiency of lipolysis and loss of body fat."[87]

Translation: Excess insulin causes weight gain and makes weight loss nearly impossible. DHEA reduces insulin levels and stimulates fat burning.

Research has also revealed a powerful synergistic effect of DHEA and resveratrol. By different but complimentary pathways, both compounds have been shown to reduce oxidative stress and improve energy metabolism.[88]

DHEA and alpha lipoic acid work together to protect the brain.[89] DHEA and Maca work together to improve libido and sexual function.[90,91] CoQ10 and DHEA synergize to improve energy levels in people with chronic fatigue.[92] Considerable research is now aimed at the synergy of DHEA, carnosine and beta alanine in life extension. Maybe some good old fashioned math equations will help drive this point home?

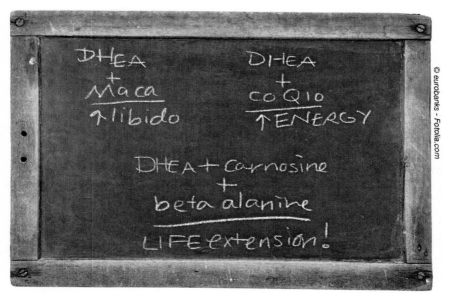

If it is such a powerful Metabolic Modifier, can it help athletic performance?

Sports organizations like the USOC and NCAA have placed DHEA on the list of banned substances. I believe that is unnecessary because, after decades of experience with hundreds of elite athletes, I have yet to see anyone "abusing" DHEA. This is because DHEA does not make you run faster or jump higher. It does not promote abnormal muscle growth. It is a repair signal, and as such, is primarily useful for preventing muscle damage during intense training.[93]

My fight with organizers of Master's level (age 50 +) competition is that virtually all competitors have low levels of DHEA compared to prime peak, and yet the supplement is still banned. In one confrontation, I asked a conference medical director if he would allow an athlete with low thyroid function to take thyroid medication. "Of course," he replied. I then asked if he could tell me the difference between an athlete taking thyroid hormone and one taking DHEA for low adrenal function. To which he replied, "Thyroid hormone is not banned, DHEA is." This is an irrational argument known as circular reasoning.

 If DHEA is such a powerful and comprehensive Metabolic Modifier, why hasn't my conventional doctor ever mentioned it to me?

DHEA is not a drug.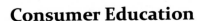

Consumer Education

While hundreds of studies have demonstrated that DHEA is a safe and effective Metabolic Modifier, one has to admit that well-controlled scientific studies are one thing, and unbridled use by the American public (motto: if a little is good, a lot is better) is something altogether different.

DHEA is a powerful hormone. It influences more than 150 metabolic functions throughout the body and brain. It's not like vitamin C, which is easily excreted in the urine. If you take too much DHEA, you can experience adverse effects.

That's because the body converts some DHEA to testosterone and estrogen, two powerful sex steroids. Thus one must be careful—something that's rather difficult to get across in a health-food store when the product is right next to the organic corn chips. I spelled out the appropriate cautions quite clearly in The DHEA Breakthrough, but still received reports of overdose symptoms such as acne, even in people who were taking a reasonable (25 to 50 mg) dose.

Some people should not take DHEA, like:

A. People under age 30 (unless following the advice of their physician). In general, young people are already producing adequate DHEA. Since the hormone can be converted to testosterone and estrogen, taking DHEA can produce symptoms associated with excess sex hormones such as acne and (in women) facial hair growth from elevated testosterone.

B. Men being treated for prostate cancer. A common medical treatment for prostate cancer is testosterone blockade, in which all sources of testosterone are suppressed. Taking DHEA in this case would be counterproductive.

C. Women being treated for breast cancer. A common medical treatment for breast cancer is estrogen blockade, with drugs like Tamoxifen™. Thus DHEA would also be counterproductive.

Easy Does It

We live in an instant-results society. However, the benefits of DHEA tend to be experienced gradually as tissue levels are optimized. Unfortunately, the hype surrounding DHEA has set up an expectation that you can take it and instantly feel 20 years younger. When this doesn't occur, people often assume they need to take more. Remember that the human body, even at age 25, produces only 40 to 70 mg of DHEA per day. A sensible replacement dose therefore should stay within that level, and research suggests that 10 to 50 mg of DHEA will be sufficient for most people.[94]

No Place for Guesswork

Natalie offers two options to her patients who need DHEA. If they are scheduled for a routine blood test, she suggests including a DHEA sulfate (DHEAS) level. Knowing how much DHEA the patient is producing (baseline) helps guide the dose recommendation. If the patient is not having blood work, she suggests starting on a low dose: 5 to 10 mg upon arising and before bed. Three to six months later, they can retest in order to find their DHEA status in the supplemented state. If still below the optimum range, they will know to increase their DHEA.

If you are taking DHEA, and want to know your DHEA status, you should TAKE your evening dose, SKIP your morning dose, and have your blood drawn before noon.

Normal vs. Optimum

Natalie note

In my entire medical career, I have only seen three patients who were not in the normal range for DHEAS. That's because the lab's reference range is likely to go from 50 to 520. You don't have to be a clinical chemist to see that this is absurd. How is it possible for one person to be normal with a DHEAS level of 50, while another person of the same age is normal at ten times that amount? What's going on?

First, let's understand that a reference range is determined by the amounts that are common in a reference group of people the same age. Since people vary widely in the amount of DHEA they produce, the "normal" range for this critical biomarker is enormous, and also meaningless.

What you really want to know is this: within this reference range spanning orders of magnitude, what is optimum? Fortunately, this can be calculated by studying published medical literature, which Stephen has been doing for more than 30 years. He is also, I believe, the oldest American scientist who has been consistently supplementing with DHEA for more than 25 years.

12. Resveratrol

If DHEA is involved in hundreds of metabolic functions throughout the body and brain, resveratrol is a close second. Derived primarily from Japanese knotweed (Polygonum cuspidatum), resveratrol is also found in grape skins, red wine and peanut butter.

Early research focused on the longevity benefits, as scientists extended the lifespan of yeast and fruit flies. But when resveratrol failed to produce the same effect in more complex organisms, interest waned. Fortunately, many scientists expanded their search—looking for metabolic benefits—and hit the jackpot. In a human clinical trial published in 2011, using a dose of 150 mg per day, scientists at Boston University documented seven key benefits (documented at the tissue, cell, and genome level) that simply cannot be ignored[95]:

1. Resveratrol improved insulin sensitivity
2. Resveratrol stimulated fat burning, especially in low-nutrient conditions (e.g., after a short fast or strenuous exercise)
3. Resveratrol reduced inflammation, leading to more efficient energy transport and utilization

4. The compound up-regulated energy production in mitochondria
5. Similar to alpha-Ketoglutaric acid, resveratrol increased Krebs cycle (energy) efficiency
6. Resveratrol caused the removal of fat from the liver and stimulated the transport of that fat to skeletal muscles for energy production
7. Resveratrol reduced blood pressure and triglycerides

New research just published: If these seven benefits are not enough, here's one more: in-vitro (test tube) research shows that resveratrol can prevent fat from accumulating in preadipocytes (immature fat cells).[96] This new anti-obesity effect may turn out to be the best yet, because it could effectively prevent the formation of new fat cells.

That is incredible! Why hasn't my conventional doctor told me about this?

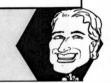

Resveratrol is not a drug.

WHEW!

We realize that this is the longest chapter, and includes the most information. So we've divided these Metabolic Modifiers into three categories: those that help you Start, those that help you Stay and those that get you Strong.

To help you START *The Metabolic Makeover*

- DHEA
- Alpha lipoic acid
- Acetyl-L-carnitine
- Resveratrol
- Alpha-Ketoglutaric acid
- Rhodiola
- Aloe
- Green tea

To help you STAY with the program and gain deeper and more significant benefits:

- Creatine
- D-Ribose
- Maca
- MCTs
- CoQ10
- Panax ginseng

To get you STRONG:

- Beta alanine
- HMB
- Cissus quadrangularis
- Leucine

Is this chapter finally over?

Not quite, because new research has revealed one more important Metabolic Modifier. To introduce this valuable and remarkably inexpensive agent, I think we need a quick review of AMPK.

You'll remember that AMPK is the primary energy sensor in the body. As cellular energy levels drop (e.g., from exercise or between meals), AMPK calls for the release of stored energy, primarily from fat. Remember our discussion of naturally thin people in Chapter 1? Their primary metabolic advantage is the ability to rapidly and efficiently burn fat. We now know that this is derived in great part from high levels of AMPK.

A detailed review in the *American Journal of Physiology* calls AMPK, "the metabolic master switch." [97] OK, so what is this new Metabolic Modifier that up-regulates AMPK?

Drum roll...

A LOW-CARBOHYDRATE DIET.

Scientists have known for decades that the life-extension benefits of calorie restriction derive in great part from up-regulation of AMPK and other signaling molecules. Now a study published in the journal, *Hormone and Metabolic Research* reveals that one does not need to restrict all calories; just carbohydrates. They conclude: "a relative deficiency in carbohydrate intake...even in the absence of caloric deprivation is sufficient to activate the AMPK-SIRT1 energy-sensing cellular network in human skeletal muscle." [98]

The last word of that paragraph is very important, leading us to the inescapable fact that all Metabolic Modifiers ultimately rely on muscle.

The Magic of Muscle

Muscle protects your joints, burns fat, strengthens bones, stimulates immunity, balances blood sugar and looks sexy. Building muscle protects against:

- Obesity
- High blood pressure
- Diabetes
- Cardiovascular disease
- Cancer
- All-cause mortality

Need I say more?

The good news is that anyone at any age, can gain and maintain muscle. But unless you are a super-fit athlete, you're going to need some help. I served on the faculty of the American College of Sports Medicine, and wrote the nutrition module for board certification in that specialty. From 1980 to 1995, I helped train Olympic athletes and world record holders in track and field, triathlon, mountaineering and martial arts. But for the last 20 years, I've been more interested in applying this experience to "normal" people.

It's rewarding to help an elite athlete win a gold medal, but Natalie and I want to help thousands of people win at life. Every one of these Metabolic Modifiers can produce measurable— sometimes astounding—results, but none of them will do any good until they are combined with exercise.

Ah, the dreaded "E" word. Isn't it interesting that so many of us flee from something that we craved when we were younger? That's because what used to be fun has become arduous and sometimes painful. Natalie and I are keenly aware of this dilemma, and have spent hundreds of hours in the lab, the clinic and the gym, to find a solution; a way to make exercise easier and more enjoyable.

We have described in this chapter how Metabolic Modifiers can improve energy, strength and stamina. These are the critical missing puzzle pieces that you need to once again exult in movement. You can call it exercise. We call it the game of life, because the human body was made to move.

Summary

1. Metabolic Modifiers are natural compounds that work by:
   - Improving energy production at the cell level
   - Increasing the body's (especially liver and muscles) ability to use fat as fuel
   - Improving glucose balance
   - Increasing exercise tolerance
   - Supporting the maintenance of high muscle mass

2. There are two modifiers (DHEA and Resveratrol) that contribute to virtually all of these pathways.

3. A low-carbohydrate diet activates many of the pathways listed above, and optimizes the benefits derived from all 30 Metabolic Modifiers.

Endnotes

1 Department of Molecular and Cell Biology, University of California, Berkeley
   * The Children's Hospital Oakland Research Institute.
   * The Department of Biochemistry and Biophysics, Linus Pauling Institute, Oregon State University, Corvallis.
   * Department of Pharmacology and Pathobiology, Royal Veterinary and Agricultural University, Copenhagen DK
   * Lawrence Berkeley national Laboratory, Berkeley, CA

2 Hagen TM, Liu J, Lykkesfeldt J, Wehr CM, Ingersoll RT, Vinarsky V, Bartholomew JC, Ames BN. Feeding acetyl-L-carnitine and lipoic acid to old rats significantly improves metabolic function while decreasing oxidative stress. Mitochondrial-supported bioenergetics decline and oxidative stress increases during aging. Proc natl Acad Sci USA. February 19, 2002;99(4):1870-1875.

3 http://www.berkeley.edu/news/berkeleyan/2002/02/27_ames.html

4 Koeth RA, Wang Z, Levison, BS, et al. Intestinal microbiota metabolism of L-carnitine, a nutrient in red meat, promotes atherosclerosis. Nature Medicine. Published online 07 April 2013. doi:10.1038/nm.3145

5 Mayo Clin Proc. Jun 2013;88(6):1-8. doi:10.1016/j.mayocp.2013.02.007.

6 Reed LJ. A trail of research from lipoic acid to alpha-keto acid dehydrogenase complexes. J Biol Chem. 2001;276(42):38329-38336.

7 Lee WJ, Song KH, Koh EH, Won JC. Alpha-lipoic acid increases insulin sensitivity by activating AMPK in skeletal muscle. Biochem Biophys Res Commun. 2005 Jul 8;332(3):885-91.

8 Gorąca A, Huk-Kolega H, Piechota A, Kleniewska P, Ciejka E, Skibska B. Lipoic acid - biological activity and therapeutic potential. Pharmacol Rep. 2011 Jul;63(4):849-58.

9 Marconi S, et al: Alpha-ketoglutarate-pyridoxine complex and human performance. Eur J Appl Physiol 1982; 49:307.

10 Liu Y, Lange R, Langanky J, Hamma T, Yang B, Steinacker JM. Improved training tolerance by supplementation with α-Keto acids in untrained young adults: a randomized, double blind, placebo-controlled trial. J Int Soc Sports Nutr. 2012 Aug 2;9(1):37. doi: 10.1186/1550-2783-9-37.

11 King DS, Baskerville R, Hellsten Y, Senchina DS, Burke LM, Stear SJ, Castell LM. A-Z of nutritional supplements: dietary supplements, sports nutrition foods and ergogenic aids for health and performance. Br J Sports Med. 2012 Jul;46(9):689-90. doi: 10.1136/bjsports-2012-091314.

12   Addis P, Shecterle LM, St Cyr JA. Cellular protection during oxidative stress: a potential role for D-ribose and antioxidants. J Diet Suppl. 2012 Sep;9(3):178-82. doi: 10.3109/19390211.2012.708715.

13   Wagner S, Herrick J, Shecterle LM, St Cyr JA. D-ribose, a metabolic substrate for congestive heart failure. Prog Cardiovasc Nurs. 2009 Jun;24(2):59-60.

14   St-Onge MP, Bourque C, Jones PJ, Ross R, Parsons WE. Medium- versus long-chain triglycerides for 27 days increases fat oxidation and energy expenditure without resulting in changes in body composition in overweight women. Int J Obes Relat Metab Disord. 2003 Jan;27(1):95-102.

15   St-Onge MP, Ross R, Parsons WD, Jones PJ. Medium-chain triglycerides increase energy expenditure and decrease adiposity in overweight men. Obes Res. 2003 Mar;11(3):395-402.

16   Nosaka N, Suzuki Y, Nagatoishi A, Kasai M, Wu J, Taguchi M.Effect of ingestion of medium-chain triacylglycerols on moderate- and high-intensity exercise in recreational athletes. J Nutr Sci Vitaminol (Tokyo). 2009 Apr;55(2):120-5.

17   Kang SI, Shin HS, Kim HM, Yoon SA, Kang SW, Kim JH, Ko HC, Kim SJ. Petalonia binghamiae extract and its constituent fucoxanthin ameliorate high-fat diet-induced obesity by activating AMP-activated protein kinase. J Agric Food Chem. 2012 Mar 8.

18   Ong KW, Hsu A, Tan BK. Anti-diabetic and anti-lipidemic effects of chlorogenic acid are mediated by AMPK activation. Biochem Pharmacol. 2013 May 1;85(9):1341-51.

19   Ong KW, Hsu A, Tan BK. Chlorogenic acid stimulates glucose transport in skeletal muscle via AMPK activation: a contributor to the beneficial effects of coffee on diabetes. PLoS One. 2012;7(3):e32718. doi: 10.1371/journal.pone.0032718.

20   Itariu BK, Zeyda M, Hochbrugger EE, Neuhofer A, et al. Long-chain n-3 PUFAs reduce adipose tissue and systemic inflammation in severely obese nondiabetic patients: a randomized controlled trial. Am J Clin Nutr. 2012 Nov;96(5):1137-49. doi: 10.3945/ajcn.112.037432.

21   Brands M, Sauerwein HP, Ackermans MT, Kersten S, Serlie MJ. Omega 3 long chain fatty acids strongly induce ANGPTL4 in humans. J Lipid Res. 2013 Jan 14.

22   Rizos EC, Ntzani EE, Bika E, Kostapanos MS, Elisaf MS. Association between omega-3 fatty acid supplementation and risk of major cardiovascular disease events: a systematic review and meta-analysis. JAMA. 2012 Sep 12;308(10):1024-33. doi: 10.1001/2012.jama.11374.

23 Krittiyawong S, Ongphiphadhanakul B, et al. Diabetes mellitus in young Thai adults. J Med Assoc Thai. 2000 Nov;83(11):1283-8.

24 Devaraj S, Yimam M, Brownell LA, Jialal I, Singh S, Jia Q. Effects of Aloe vera supplementation in subjects with prediabetes/metabolic syndrome. Metab Syndr Relat Disord. 2013 Feb;11(1):35-40. doi: 10.1089/met.2012.0066.

25 Choi HC, Kim SJ, Son KY, Oh BJ, Cho BL. Metabolic effects of aloe vera gel complex in obese prediabetes and early non-treated diabetic patients: Randomized controlled trial. Nutrition. 2013 Sep;29(9):1110-4. doi: 10.1016/j.nut.2013.02.015.

26 Anderson RA, et al: Chromium intake, absorption and excretion of subjects consuming self-selected diets. Am J Clin Nutr 1985; 41:1177-83.

27 A scientific review: the role of chromium in insulin resistance. Diabetes Educ. 2004;Suppl:2-14.

28 Wilson BE, Gondy A. Effects of chromium supplementation on fasting insulin levels and lipid parameters in healthy, non-obese young subjects. . Diabetes Res Clin Pract. 1995 Jun;28(3):179-84.

29 Barrio DA, Etcheverry SB. Potential use of vanadium compounds in therapeutics. Curr Med Chem. 2010;17(31):3632-42.

30 Judy WV, Hari SP, Stogsdill WW, Judy JS, Naguib YM, Passwater R. Antidiabetic activity of a standardized extract from Lagerstroemia speciosa leaves in Type II diabetics. A dose-dependence study. J Ethnopharmacol. 2003 Jul;87(1):115-7.

31 2. Liu F, Kim J, Li Y, Liu X, Li J, Chen X. An extract of Lagerstroemia speciosa L. has insulin-like glucose uptake-stimulatory and adipocyte differentiation-inhibitory activities in 3T3-L1 cells. J Nutr. 2001 Sep;131(9):2242-7.

32 Dong H, Wang N, Zhao L, Lu F. Berberine in the treatment of type 2 diabetes mellitus: a systemic review and meta-analysis. Evid Based Complement Alternat Med. 2012;2012:591-654. doi: 10.1155/2012/591654.

33 Lee YS, Kim WS, Kim KH, et al. Berberine, a Natural Plant Product, Activates AMPK With Beneficial Metabolic Effects in Diabetic and Insulin-Resistant States. Diabetes 2013; 62(8).

34 Tian J, Dang HN, Yong J, Chui W-S, Dizon MPG, et al. (2011) Oral Treatment with γ-Aminobutyric Acid Improves Glucose Tolerance and Insulin Sensitivity by Inhibiting Inflammation in High Fat Diet-Fed Mice. PLoS ONE 6(9): e25338. doi:10.1371/journal.pone.0025338

35 Han K, Shin IC, Choi KJ, Yun YP, Hong JT, Oh KW. Korea red ginseng water extract increases nitric oxide concentrations in exhaled breath. Nitric Oxide. 2005 May;12(3):159-62.

36 Kim HG, Cho JH, Yoo SR, Lee JS, Han JM, Lee NH, Ahn YC, Son CG. Antifatigue effects of Panax ginseng C.A. Meyer: a randomised, double-blind, placebo-controlled trial. PLoS One. 2013 Apr 17;8(4):e61271. doi: 10.1371/journal.pone.0061271.

37 Vuksan V, Sung MK, Sievenpiper JL, Stavro PM, Jenkins AL, Di Buono M, Lee KS, Leiter LA, Nam KY, Arnason JT, Choi M, Naeem A. Korean red ginseng (Panax ginseng) improves glucose and insulin regulation in well-controlled, type 2 diabetes: results of a randomized, double-blind, placebo-controlled study of efficacy and safety. Nutr Metab Cardiovasc Dis. 2008 Jan;18(1):46-56.

38 Dong GZ, Jang EJ, Kang SH, Cho IJ, Park SD, Kim SC, Kim YW.Red ginseng abrogates oxidative stress via mitochondria protection mediated by LKB1-AMPK pathway. BMC Complement Altern Med. 2013 Mar 18;13:64. doi: 10.1186/1472-6882-13-64..

39 Ramesh T, Kim SW, Hwang SY, Sohn SH, Yoo SK, Kim SK. Panax ginseng reduces oxidative stress and restores antioxidant capacity in aged rats. Nutr Res. 2012 Sep;32(9):718-26. doi: 10.1016/j.nutres.2012.08.005.

40 Ye R, Kong X, Yang Q, Zhang Y, Han J, Zhao G. Ginsenoside Rd attenuates redox imbalance and improves stroke outcome after focal cerebral ischemia in aged mice. Neuropharmacology. 2011 Sep;61(4):815-24. doi: 10.1016/j.neuropharm.2011.05.029.

41 Chen F, Chen Y, Kang X, Zhou Z, Zhang Z, Liu D. Anti-apoptotic function and mechanism of ginseng saponins in Rattus pancreatic β-cells. Biol Pharm Bull. 2012;35(9):1568-73.

42 Hong B, Ji YH, Hong JH, Nam KY, Ahn TY. A double-blind crossover study evaluating the efficacy of korean red ginseng in patients with erectile dysfunction: a preliminary report. J Urol. 2002 Nov;168(5):2070-3.

43 Price A, Gazewood J. Korean red ginseng effective for treatment of erectile dysfunction. J Fam Pract. 2003 Jan;52(1):20-1.

44 http://www.itmonline.org/arts/quintozene.htm

45 Stull AJ, Cash KC, Johnson WD, Champagne CM, Cefalu WT. Bioactives in blueberries improve insulin sensitivity in obese, insulin-resistant men and women. J Nutr. 2010 Oct;140(10):1764-8. doi: 10.3945/jn.110.125336.

46 Wedick NM, Pan A, Cassidy A, Rimm EB, Sampson L, Rosner B, Willett W, Hu FB, Sun Q, van Dam RM. Dietary flavonoid intakes and risk of type 2 diabetes in US men and women. Am J Clin Nutr. 2012 Apr;95(4):925-33. doi: 10.3945/ajcn.111.028894.

47 Etzel MR (2004). "Manufacture and use of dairy protein fractions". The Journal of Nutrition 134 (4): 996S–1002S. PMID 15051860

48 L. Combaret, et al. Human Nutrition Research Centre of Clermont-Ferrand. "A leucine-supplemented diet restores the defective postprandial inhibition of proteasome-dependent proteolysis in aged rat skeletal muscle". Journal of Physiology Volume 569, issue 2, p. 489-499. Retrieved 2008-03-25.

49 Norton LE, Wilson GJ, Layman DK, Moulton CJ, Garlick PJ. Leucine content of dietary proteins is a determinant of postprandial skeletal muscle protein synthesis in adult rats. Nutrition & Metabolism 2012, 9:67 doi:10.1186/1743-7075-9-67

50 Burke, Darren G.; Chilibeck, Philip D.; Parise, Gianni; Tarnopolsky, Mark A.; Candow, Darren G. (2003). "Effect of α-Lipoic Acid Combined With Creatine Monohydrate on Human Skeletal Muscle Creatine and Phosphagen Concentration". International Journal of Sport Nutrition and Exercise Metabolism 13 (3): 294–302. PMID 14669930.

51 Bae ON, Serfozo K, Baek SH, Lee KY, Dorrance A, Rumbeiha W, Fitzgerald SD, Farooq MU, Naravelta B, Bhatt A, Majid A. Safety and efficacy evaluation of carnosine, an endogenous neuroprotective agent for ischemic stroke. Stroke. 2013 Jan;44(1):205-12. doi: 10.1161/STROKEAHA.112.673954

52 Boldyrev AA. Carnosine: new concept for the function of an old molecule. Biochemistry (Mosc). 2012 Apr;77(4):313-26. doi: 10.1134/S0006297912040013.

53 Reddy, V. P.; Garrett, MR; Perry, G; Smith, MA (2005). "Carnosine: A Versatile Antioxidant and Antiglycating Agent". Science of Aging Knowledge Environment 2005 (18): pe12. doi:10.1126/sageke.2005.18.pe12. PMID 15872311.

54 Stellingwerff T, Decombaz J, Harris RC, Boesch C. Optimizing human in vivo dosing and delivery of β-alanine supplements for muscle carnosine synthesis. Amino Acids. 2012 Jul;43(1):57-65. doi: 10.1007/s00726-012-1245-7. Epub 2012 Feb 23.

55 Everaert I, Stegen S, Vanheel B, Taes Y, Derave W. Effect of beta-alanine and carnosine supplementation on muscle contractility in mice. Med Sci Sports Exerc. 2013 Jan;45(1):43-51. doi: 10.1249/MSS.0b013e31826cdb68.

56 Harris RC, Sale C. Beta-alanine supplementation in high-intensity exercise. Med Sport Sci. 2012;59:1-17. doi: 10.1159/000342372. Epub 2012 Oct 15.

57 Sale C, Hill CA, Ponte J, Harris RC. β-alanine supplementation improves isometric endurance of the knee extensor muscles. J Int Soc Sports Nutr. 2012 Jun 14;9(1):26. doi: 10.1186/1550-2783-9-26.

58 Muthusami S, Senthilkumar K, Vignesh C, Ilangovan R, Stanley J, Selvamurugan N, Srinivasan N. Effects of Cissus quadrangularis on the proliferation, differentiation and matrix mineralization of human osteoblast like SaOS-2 cells. J Cell Biochem. 2011 Apr;112(4):1035-45. doi: 10.1002/jcb.23016.

59 Hasani-Ranjbar S, Nayebi N, Larijani B, Abdollahi M.A systematic review of the efficacy and safety of herbal medicines used in the treatment of obesity. World J Gastroenterol. 2009 Jul 7;15(25):3073-85.

60 Oben JE, Enyegue DM, Fomekong GI, Soukontoua YB, Agbor GA. The effect of Cissus quadrangularis (CQR-300) and a Cissus formulation (CORE) on obesity and obesity-induced oxidative stress. Lipids Health Dis. 2007 Feb 4;6:4.

61 Chidambaram J, Carani Venkatraman A. Cissus quadrangularis stem alleviates insulin resistance, oxidative injury and fatty liver disease in rats fed high fat plus fructose diet. Food Chem Toxicol. 2010 Aug-Sep;48(8-9):2021-9.

62 Gallagher PM, Carrithers JA, Godard MP, Schulze KE, Trappe SW. Beta-hydroxy-beta-methylbutyrate ingestion, Part I: effects on strength and fat free mass. Med Sci Sports Exerc. 2000 Dec;32(12):2109-15.

63 Knitter AE, Panton L, Rathmacher JA, Petersen A, Sharp R. Effects of beta-hydroxy-beta-methylbutyrate on muscle damage after a prolonged run. J Appl Physiol. 2000 Oct;89(4):1340-4.

64 Zanchi NE, Gerlinger-Romero F, Guimarães-Ferreira L, de Siqueira Filho MA, Felitti V, Lira FS, Seelaender M, Lancha AH Jr. HMB supplementation: clinical and athletic performance-related effects and mechanisms of action. Amino Acids. 2011 Apr;40(4):1015-25. doi: 10.1007/s00726-010-0678-0.

65 Stone M, Ibarra A, Roller M, Zangara A, Stevenson E. A pilot investigation into the effect of maca supplementation on physical activity and sexual desire in sportsmen. J Ethnopharmacol. 2009 Dec 10;126(3):574-6. doi: 10.1016/j.jep.2009.09.012.

66 Večeřa R, Orolin J, et al. The Influence of Maca (Lepidium meyenii) on Antioxidant Status, Lipid and Glucose Metabolism in Rat. Plant Foods Hum Nutr. 2007 Feb 27.

67 Choi, EH, Kang J Il, Cho JY, et al. Supplementation of standardized lipid-soluble extract from maca (Lepidium meyenii) increases swimming endurance capacity in rats. Journal of Functional Foods, Volume 4, issue 2 (April, 2012), p. 568-573

68 Li HB, Ge YK, Zheng XX, Zhang L. Salidroside stimulated glucose uptake in skeletal muscle cells by activating AMP-activated protein kinase. Eur J Pharmacol. 2008 Apr 20.

69 Noreen EE, Buckley JG, Lewis SL, Brandauer J, Stuempfle KJ. The Effects of an Acute Dose of Rhodiola Rosea on Endurance Exercise Performance. J Strength Cond Res. 2012 May 24.

70 Parisi A, Tranchita E, Duranti G, Ciminelli E, Quaranta F, Ceci R, Cerulli C, Borrione P, Sabatini S. Effects of chronic Rhodiola Rosea supplementation on sport performance and antioxidant capacity in trained male: preliminary results. J Sports Med Phys Fitness. 2010 Mar;50(1):57-63.

71 De Bock K, Eijnde BO, Ramaekers M, Hespel P. Acute Rhodiola rosea intake can improve endurance exercise performance. Int J Sport Nutr Exerc Metab. 2004 Jun;14(3):298-307.

72 Lukaski HC, Nielsen FH. Dietary Magnesium Depletion Affects Metabolic Responses during Submaximal Exercise in Postmenopausal Women. J. Nutr. May 1, 2002 vol. 132 no. 5 930-935

73 Lucotti P, Setola E, Monti LD, et al. Beneficial effects of a long-term oral L-arginine added to a hypocaloric diet and exercise training program in obese, insulin-resistant type-2 diabetic patients. Am J Physiol Endocrinol Metab 2006; 291:E906-E912.

74 McKnight JR, Satterfield MC, Jobgen W, et al. Beneficial effects of L-arginine on reducing obesity: potential mechanisms and important implications for human health. Amino Acids 2010; 39:349-357.

75 Olson RE, Rudney H: Biosynthesis of ubiquinone. Vitamins and hormones 1983; 40:2-43.

76 Choi M, Park H, Cho S, Lee M. Vitamin D3 supplementation modulates inflammatory responses from the muscle damage induced by high-intensity exercise in SD rats. Cytokine 2013, May 10. http://www.sciencedirect.com/science/article/pii/S1043466613001373

77 Orentreich N, Brind JL, Vogelman JH, Andres R, Baldwin H. Long-term longitudinal measurements of plasma dehydro-epiandrosterone sulfate in normal men. J Clin Endocrinol Metab 1992; 75: 1002-1004.

78 Kichigin VA, Markova TN, Madianov IV, Semakina SM, Borisova LV, Bashkova IB. Adaptive systems of the body in metabolic syndrome. Klin Med (Mosk). 2012;90(8):50-4.

79   Villareal DT, Holloszy JO, Kohrt WM. Effects of DHEA replacement on bone mineral density and body composition in elderly women and men. Clin Endocrinol (Oxf) 2000 Nov;53(5):561-8

80   Kawano H, Yasue H, Kitagawa A, Hirai N, Yoshida T, Soejima H, Miyamoto S, Nakano M, Ogawa H. Dehydroepiandrosterone supplementation improves endothelial function and insulin sensitivity in men. J Clin Endocrinol Metab. 2003 Jul;88(7):3190-5.

81   Villareal DT, Holloszy JO. Effect of DHEA on Abdominal Fat and Insulin Action in Elderly Women and Men. A Randomized Controlled Trial. JAMA. 2004;292(18):2243-2248. doi:10.1001/jama. 292.18.2243.

82   Weiss EP, Villareal DT, Fontana L, Han DH, Holloszy JO. Dehydroepiandrosterone (DHEA) replacement decreases insulin resistance and lowers inflammatory cytokines in aging humans. Aging (Albany NY). 2011 May;3(5):533-42.

83   Dumas de La Roque E, Baulieu EÉ, et al. Dehydroepiandrosterone (DHEA) improves pulmonary hypertension in chronic obstructive pulmonary disease (COPD): a pilot study. Ann Endocrinol (Paris). 2012 Feb;73(1):20-5. doi: 10.1016/j.ando.2011.12.005.

84   Huang YJ, Chen MT, Fang CL, Lee WC, Yang SC, Kuo CH. A possible link between exercise-training adaptation and dehydroepiandrosterone sulfate- an oldest-old female study. Int J Med Sci. 2006 Sep 10;3(4):141-7.

85   Bloch M, Schmidt PJ, Danaceau MA, Adams LF, Rubinow DR. Dehydroepiandrosterone treatment of midlife dysthymia. Biol Psychiatry 1999 Jun 15;45(12):1533-41

86   Chiu KM, Schmidt MJ, Havighurst TC, Shug AL, Daynes RA, Keller ET, Gravenstein S. Correlation of serum L-carnitine and dehydro-epi-androsterone sulphate levels with age and sex in healthy adults. Age Ageing 1999 Mar;28(2):211-6

87   Pergola GD. The adipose tissue metabolism: role of testosterone and DHEA. Int J Obesity 2000; 24: Suppl 2. S59-S-63

88   Mousa SA, Gallati C, Simone T, Dier E, Yalcin M, Dyskin E, Thangirala S, Hanko C, Rebbaa A. Dual targeting of the antagonistic pathways mediated by Sirt1 and TXNIP as a putative approach to enhance the efficacy of anti-aging interventions. Aging (Albany NY). 2009 Mar 31;1(4):412-24.

89   Sinha M, Saha A, Basu S, Pal K, Chakrabarti S. Aging and antioxidants modulate rat brain levels of homocysteine and DHEA sulphate (DHEA-S): implications in the pathogenesis of Alzheimer's disease. Neurosci Lett. 2010 Oct 11;483(2):123-6. doi: 10.1016/j.neulet.2010.07.075.

90 McKay D. Nutrients and botanicals for erectile dysfunction: examining the evidence. Altern Med Rev. 2004 Mar;9(1):4-16.

91 Balick MJ, Lee R. Maca: from traditional food crop to energy and libido stimulant. Altern Ther Health Med. 2002 Mar-Apr;8(2):96-8.

92 Bentler SE, Hartz AJ, Kuhn EM. Prospective observational study of treatments for unexplained chronic fatigue. J Clin Psychiatry. 2005 May;66(5):625-32.

93 Liao YH, Liao KF, Kao CL, Chen CY, Huang CY, Chang WH, Ivy JL, Bernard JR, Lee SD, Kuo CH. Effect of dehydroepiandrosterone administration on recovery from mix-type exercise training-induced muscle damage. Eur J Appl Physiol. 2013 Jan;113(1):99-107. doi: 10.1007/s00421-012-2409-6.

94 P.R. Casson, A. Morales and J.E. Buster. The use and effects of DHEA in humans. in: DHEA: A Comprehensive Review. J.H.H. Thijssen and H. Nieuwenhuyse (eds.) New York, Parthenon, 1999. Pg 127-152.

95 Timmers S, Konings E, Bilet L, et al. Calorie Restriction-like Effects of 30 Days of Resveratrol Supplementation on Energy Metabolism and Metabolic Profile in Obese Humans. Cell Metabolism 14, 612–622, November 2, 2011

96 Mol Nutr Food Res. 2012 Sep 4. doi: 10.1002/mnfr.201100772. Delipidating effect of resveratrol metabolites in 3T3-L1 adipocytes. Lasa A, Churruca I, Eseberri I, Andrés-Lacueva C, Portillo MP.

97 Winder WW, Hardie DG: AMP-activated protein kinase, a metabolic master switch: possible roles in type 2 diabetes. Am J Physiol 1999; 277:E1–E10

98 Draznin B, Wang C, Adochio R, Leitner JW, Cornier MA. Effect of dietary macronutrient composition on AMPK and SIRT1 expression and activity in human skeletal muscle. Horm Metab Res. 2012 Sep;44(9):650-5. doi: 10.1055/s-0032-1312656.

REFLECTIONS

---

1. Have you ever started an exercise program and quit?

2. Did you blame yourself?

3. Do you see now that Metabolic Modifiers were the missing puzzle piece?

4. Which Metabolic Modifiers appeal to you? Where do you place yourself? Start, Stay or Get Strong?

Notes:

Chapter Nine

ENERGY

"NFL Football. 22 players in desperate need of rest, being watched by 22 million spectators in desperate need of exercise."

We were going to call this the "Exercise Chapter," but if we did, many readers would skip it, in the same way that they avoid exercise. But by calling it the "Energy Chapter," we hope to trick more people into reading it.

After all, the terms *exercise* and *energy* are actually synonymous. And I'm not talking about how exercise *requires* energy. It is far more important to understand that exercise *creates* energy.

Everybody wants more energy. This entire book is about energy. Natalie's medical practice and my career as a scientist are devoted — in great part — to maximizing cellular energy. That's because energy drives repair and optimal repair confers the highest possible quality of life.

OK picture this: you're hired as a vice president by a large corporation. You do an excellent job and expect a bonus at the end of the year. You open your envelope to find a check for $5,000. A little disappointed, you ask your colleague, also a VP hired on the same day, what she received. Beaming, she shows you a check for $200,000! Think that's fair? Would you be outraged and demand an explanation? Of course.

But lets take the analogy a bit further. What happens when your colleague leaves for home? I want you to imagine her mood as she steps into the elevator. She is radiating joy. Then in the parking lot, how do you think she is feeling as she inserts her key into the door of the car she is about to trade in for a BMW 750?

Many of you probably know that I'm not talking about money, but rather the currency of LIFE, known as cellular energy. And in fact, it is quite possible for one person to have a modicum of energy, and for someone else to have 40 TIMES that amount. True, part of it is genetic. You know that the children of thin, athletic parents are born with a metabolic advantage. But you also know now that DNA is not destiny, and that *The Metabolic Makeover* creates a level playing field. Everyone has the same chance for the big bonus.

Do you aspire to be average?

How do you think someone making 40 times the energy of an average person feels? How do they move through life? What thoughts do they think? I can assure you, it is not an average life by any measure; and so it is astounding to me that this is still not clearly understood by the vast majority of people who are sucking down "energy drinks" and wondering why they wake up feeling like they've been hit by a bus.

High-energy people bound out of bed. They don't need alarm clocks because even their sleep is deeper and more rejuvenating than the average sedentary person. So they wake up refreshed and eager to move into the day.

You may be wondering why fit people have higher quality (more rejuvenating) sleep compared to unfit people. Again, it has to do with muscles. We're all extremely busy, so everyone's brain is tired by the time 11:00 p.m. rolls around. But here's the sedentary person's 11:15 p.m.

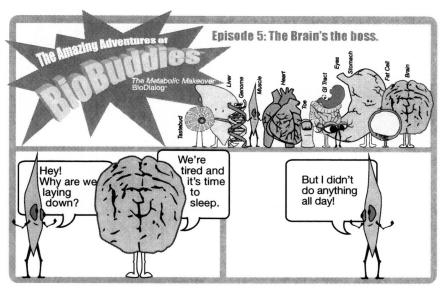

You see the dilemma. Deep sleep is triggered primarily by tired muscles. Sedentary people rarely have tired muscles. I've seen clients who reported with amazement, that over the weekend they helped a friend move; and that night, they "slept better than they have in years." I would then inform them that they don't have to wait for a friend to move. They can enjoy that deep, rejuvenating sleep every night. It's a choice.

Where did you get the 40X figure?

That's an estimate, based on increased glycogen and mitochondrial density. In Chapter 3, you learned that glycogen is an energy storage compound in the muscles and liver. You might remember that an active person will have about 20 times the glycogen storage as a sedentary person, and an elite athlete could double that. In other words, 40 times the glycogen storage compared to a sedentary person of the same size.

In Chapter 8, we described mitochondria as the "energy factories" within each cell. When muscles are worked, they require more energy, so new mitochondria are formed. Moreover, all the mitochondria become more efficient. A muscle cell from a fit person can have more than ten times the mitochondria compared to an unfit person. Then multiply that by an unknown (but significant) factor based on the fact that a fit person can have a few hundred billion more muscle cells... 40 times actually may be conservative.

When all is said and done, it's not about numbers, is it? It's about how you look and feel. Natalie and I have both seen — with thousands of clients — how adding muscle **c h a n g e s e v e r y t h i n g .** First, there's the physical sense of being more capable. And then there's the emotional sense associated with being strong. You put those together, and clients have used words like invincible. How would you like to feel invincible?

A woman came up to me at a conference and thanked me for changing her life. "How'd that happen?" I asked. She explained that she was a psychology professor, and the entrance to the social sciences building was one of those huge metal doors. Every day, as she approached the door, she would hold her books with both arms—even if she only had a few books or even just one book— and wait for a student to open the door.

After about 6 weeks on *The Metabolic Makeover*, she strode up to the door, flung a pile of books under one arm, reached for the huge door handle and was half-way through the entrance when she gasped with a life-changing realization.

She realized that her past self-image had been that of a powerless woman. In a flash, she saw what was missing in her life; and it wasn't more degrees or academic awards. It was physical strength. And the addition of a little muscle in her arms, shoulders, and chest was the tipping point to a new sense of who she was. That enabled her to end an abusive relationship and embrace a part of life that had actually frightened her in the past.

As an awkward "nerdy" young girl, she was teased and harassed by boys. So like many, she retreated into her mind, where she knew she could excel. But her genome was not going for that. Certainly, a sharp mind was a valuable asset. For 2 million years, however, survival depended primarily on strength and agility. Thus, standing as we are in the 21st century, but defined in great part by ancient DNA, we cannot forget what got us this far; a balance of mental, emotional, and physical strength. Without this balance you simply cannot feel invincible.

How do you feel right now, at this moment?

That's right. I'd like you to put this book down for a few minutes and take a quick inventory of your state. Do you feel energetic, strong, and relaxed? Are there parts of your body that you would like to strengthen? Would you like to lose weight? Are you feeling excited and optimistic about the future?

Take a deep breath and know, in your core, that all of these things are possible. No matter how many times you have tried and failed; no matter your age or physical condition, you can rebuild and rejuvenate 300 billion cells a day, and create the life you want. Now, if you've been sedentary for a decade or more, you may not remember what vitality feels like. So here's a tip: raise the bar an inch at a time.

When I was working with Olympic track and field athletes, I was surprised to see the way high jumpers practice. There were athletes on that team who could easily clear seven feet. But they would start with the bar at around six feet, and with each successive jump, as they warmed up, they would raise the bar an inch or two. Then at seven feet, they would raise it half an inch at a time.

This is how to rebuild your body. Don't set the bar at a world-record height. Don't compare yourself to others. Set the bar where you know you can succeed then raise it a few inches at a time.

Here's another lesson I learned from high-jumpers. Nothing is accomplished if you don't raise the bar. How many people do you know who are in exercise ruts—sometimes for years—where they run 30 minutes on a treadmill and do three machines at the same resistance for the same number of reps. They maintain a modicum of fitness, but miss out on the tremendous energy, strength, and vitality that comes when you challenge yourself.

The Bottom Line

1. It's all about energy
2. More muscle = more energy
3. More energy = more repair
4. More repair = greater quality of life

...AND MOST LIKELY, A **L O N G E R** LIFE.

I call this the Jack LaLanne effect. Evidence strongly suggests that muscle mass is not only important, it appears to be the primary factor determining your longevity. Recently, researchers discovered an entire class of repair-and-rebuild signaling molecules derived from muscle. These myokines, according to one study, "modulate systemic physiology" meaning that they control repair functions throughout the body.[1]

> The only way to build and maintain muscle is to exercise.

Why do so few people exercise on a regular basis?

Excuses.

OK. Call them *obstacles*.

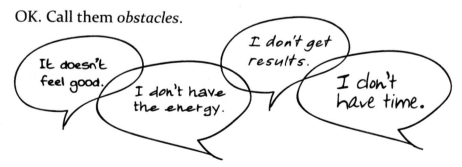

Every day, Natalie and I see people overcoming the first three obstacles by using Metabolic Modifiers from Chapter 8 alone. To a great extent, these obstacles all relate to a single factor: AGING.

You see, as we lose the anabolic (build/repair) metabolism of youth, we lose muscle mass. Decreased muscle mass (and muscle quality) means fewer mitochondria (energy factories) and dramatically reduced glycogen stores. Thus, our bodies begin to interpret exercise as stress. This shift increases the production of the catabolic (wear down, break down) hormone cortisol, which lowers DHEA, suppresses immunity, and contributes to a number of degenerative problems, not to mention weight gain. Clearly, this vicious cycle must be reversed.

DHEA. Again.

If I didn't drive this message (the importance of DHEA) home enough before, here I go again. Optimizing DHEA can restore healthy anabolic metabolism. DHEA also raises levels of a repair biochemical known as Insulin-Like Growth Factor 1 (IGF-1). This can decrease your recovery time after a workout and dramatically improve muscle repair and synthesis.[2]

Gerontologists have known for decades that IGF-1 decreases as we age, but they accepted this decrease as an irreversible result of the aging process. We now know that IGF-1 levels can be restored.

Researchers gave DHEA to a group of men in their late fifties. After only 30 days, they documented a remarkable 90% increase in IGF-1.[3] This translates into greater muscle growth and maintenance for anyone over 35. Furthermore, Natalie reports that this benefit is even more pronounced in her female patients.

Look good in your genes

Another benefit of DHEA supplementation is a marked improvement in muscle definition soon after beginning a strength-training program. An excellent study reported in the *Annals of the New York Academy of Sciences* concluded:

> DHEA in appropriate replacement doses appears to have remedial effects with respect to its ability to induce an anabolic growth factor, increase muscle strength and lean body mass, activate immune function, and enhance quality of life in aging men and women, with no significant adverse effects.
>
> YEN SS, MORALES AJ, KHORRAM O. REPLACEMENT OF DHEA IN AGING MEN AND WOMEN. POTENTIAL REMEDIAL EFFECTS. ANN NY ACAD SCI, 1995 DEC 29, 774:128-42..

Clearly, if you're over 35, DHEA is the key to metabolic and physical fitness. It's not a magic bullet, but without it, your chance of success is greatly reduced.

Natalie note

It astounds me that 18 years after Stephen wrote The DHEA Breakthrough and more than 7,000 published studies later, I still encounter health professionals who are entirely unfamiliar with this critically important Metabolic Modifier. Everyone should measure their DHEA sulfate (DHEAS) level at their annual physical. However, since it is not included in a standard blood chemistry, you will have to ask for it. I have found a review article that may help if you need to explain to your doctor why you want this information. In fact, you should only need this concluding statement:

> "DHEA modulates endothelial function, reduces inflammation, improves insulin sensitivity, blood flow, cellular immunity, body composition, bone metabolism, sexual function, and physical strength in frailty and provides neuroprotection, improves cognitive function, and memory enhancement. DHEA possesses

pleiotropic effects and reduced levels of DHEA and
DHEA-S may be associated with a host of pathologies."

TRAISH AM, KANG HP, SAAD F, GUAY AT DEHYDROEPIANDROSTE-
RONE (DHEA)-A PRECURSOR STEROID OR AN ACTIVE HORMONE IN
HUMAN PHYSIOLOGY (CME). J SEX MED. 2011 NOV;8(11):2960-2982.
DOI: 10.1111/J.1743-6109.2011.02523.X.

The Opportunity of a Lifetime

With DHEA and other Metabolic Modifiers, we find ourselves standing on the threshold of a new era which will enable us to move beyond the constraints and limitations of evolution. Muscle really is magic, and the most amazing muscle in your body is beating inside your chest.

Picture this: you are passing a pet store window, and there is the most adorable dog you have ever seen. The shop owner explains that, while this breed of dog can be the most amazing companion imaginable, they have very specific dietary and exercise needs. Failing to provide premium nutrition or daily activity will dramatically reduce the lifespan of this beautiful animal. Most people would be more than willing to do that in order to maintain the health of a beautiful dog. Why is it that so few understand that the human heart has the same requirements?

The Heart of the Matter

Researchers at Baylor School of Medicine wanted to study the effect of education on health outcomes. They chose heart-attack survivors, creating two groups, matched for age and weight. One group got the recommended drugs, as well as diet and lifestyle counseling. The second group received the same, along with a two-hour course on "how the heart works." Over the next 5 years, the group that got the two-hour education suffered one third fewer heart attacks.

IF PEOPLE *KNEW* BETTER, THEY'D *DO* BETTER.

It's useful to think of your heart and lungs as a single, integrated structure. Scientists call this the cardiorespiratory system, which is responsible for extracting oxygen from the air you breathe and then transporting that oxygen to 75 trillion cells from the top of your head to the tips of your toes.

To a great extent, oxygen = energy, and as we know, repeat after me: **"It's All About Energy."** Thus, anyone desiring a long and healthy life should put cardiorespiratory fitness at the top of their "to-do" list.

The heart, of course, is a muscle, and like other muscles, requires exercise to maintain optimal function. Importantly, the operation of the lungs also depends upon a series of muscles that move air in and out. When those muscles decondition (through lack of exercise), respiratory fitness declines and cells start to suffocate.

Really, "suffocate?"

Well, the scientific term is hypoxia, but most people don't know that word and this is an important point. Cellular health and energy production is a continuum from optimum to cell death. We're trying to emphasize the fact that insufficient oxygen delivery reduces cellular health and energy production. Depending on the cell type, this can dramatically reduce your quality of life. The process is completely silent until a critical event takes place, such as a heart attack, kidney failure, or a stroke.

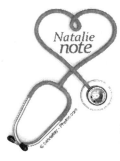

Natalie note

During a physical exam, I pay close attention to the appearance of the patient's feet. Color, temperature and pulse tell me a lot about oxygen delivery to the extremities. I used to think that this was age-related, but I have noticed that even young people can have poor circulation, indicating low metabolic fitness.

Get a Move On

No matter where you are right now, you can experience dramatic cardiorespiratory improvements in as little as 6 weeks. Some you will feel, while other benefits will be just as important but silent. Here's what you can expect from a sensible and consistent exercise program:

1. Your heart gets stronger
2. It may even increase in size
3. Increase in size and volume of the ventricular chambers
4. Increased stroke volume; meaning that every beat of your heart sends more oxygen to your cells.
5. With consistent exercise, the capillary density of the heart muscle increases, meaning greater blood flow to the heart itself.
6. Increased supply of blood and oxygen allows the heart to beat more strongly and efficiently during rest and exercise.

English please.

The right ventricle chamber sends blood to the lungs. The left ventricle sends oxygenated blood throughout the body.

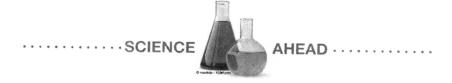
How does this translate to vastly improved metabolic efficiency?

To deliver oxygen to every cell of your body, your heart has to pump about five liters of blood per minute. Thus, circulation (C) can be calculated as stroke volume (SV) multiplied by heart rate (HR).

C = SV x HR

So what happens when you increase your cardio fitness, and your stroke volume increases? Since C is a constant 5 liters/minute, your heart does not have to beat as fast to deliver those 5 liters of blood.

This is where we talk about resting heart rate and what an important indicator it is for measuring metabolic efficiency. Using the simple equation C=SV x HR, the average person's situation looks like this: **5L/min = 70 mL/beat x 72 beats/min**

A fit individual, however, will have a stroke volume close to 100. That means with every beat, the heart pumps out 100 mL of blood instead of 70, so the number of heart beats (resting heart rate) will decline **5L/min = 100 mL/beat x 50 beats/min**

The heart of an elite athlete may be so strong that every beat pumps out close to 150 mL of blood. Thus it is not unusual for a superfit individual to have a resting heart rate of 35 beats per minute.

The Bottom Line

That means, on an average day, an unfit person's heart has to beat 31,680 times more than a fit person. And compared to an endurance athlete, the unfit person's heart must beat an additional 53,280 times—every day—just to get oxygen to their cells. Over the course of a year, that comes to more than 19 million extra beats. **W h e w !**

Exercise tolerance

We all have excuses why we don't exercise, but one of the most common complaints I heard in clinical practice was, "it doesn't feel good." This highlights the biggest Catch-22 in the quest for peak health: you can't be fit unless you exercise, but you can't really enjoy exercise unless you're fit. What to do?

Start where you are and build up slowly. My favorite definition of exercise is: "Being more active today than you were yesterday." More activity—no matter what kind of activity—will improve cardiorespiratory efficiency. And with the help of Metabolic Modifiers, that can occur rapidly. Here's how.

When muscles contract during exercise, they send a message to the heart and lungs, "more oxygen please!" The unfit person's cardiorespiratory system is slow to respond, so the muscles rapidly tire and get sore. But with consistent exercise and Metabolic Modifiers to speed conversion of fat into energy, the response time improves and exercise starts to feel good. Building up to strenuous exercise like power walking, the average man or woman can nearly double their cardiac output.

Another factor in exercise tolerance is recovery time. That's the time it takes for your heart, lungs and blood vessels to restore oxygen levels and remove metabolic waste. With consistent exercise, you'll notice that your heart rate will return to normal much faster, leaving you feeling invigorated, not exhausted.

The subtitle of this book is, "It's all about energy." We've covered a lot of energy physiology, including the role of glycogen, mitochondrial density, how to increase the number and strength of muscle cells, the importance of fat-burning metabolic pathways, the problem of insulin resistance, and the fact that aging is accompanied by decreased circulation throughout the body and brain.

Every one of these factors is improved with exercise. Nothing else works long term, which is why Natalie and I are so devoted to helping you get moving.

BUT WAIT...THERE'S MORE!

You don't breathe oxygen. You breathe air, which is only about 21% oxygen. Structures within your lungs known as alveoli extract oxygen from inhaled air, and this process (pulmonary diffusion) is enhanced by exercise.

That oxygen is carried to the cells by a compound in red blood cells known as hemoglobin. Exercise can increase both the number of red blood cells and their hemoglobin content.

The bloodstream delivers oxygen to the cells through narrow blood vessels known as capillaries. Exercise can increase the number of capillaries supplying each muscle fiber by as much as 50%.

To get through these incredibly narrow capillaries, the blood needs to be rather "thin." Exercise reduces the fat content of the blood (triglycerides and cholesterol), improves blood viscosity, and raises cardio-protective HDL.

Myoglobin is a substance in the muscle cell that attracts oxygen from the bloodstream into the muscle. Exercise increases myoglobin stores.

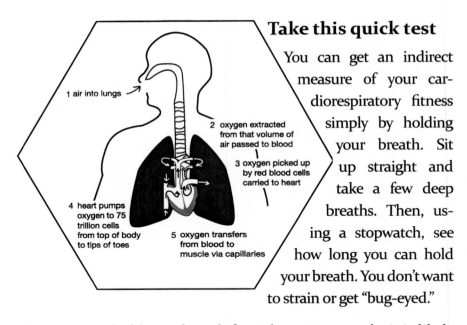

1 air into lungs

2 oxygen extracted from that volume of air passed to blood

3 oxygen picked up by red blood cells carried to heart

4 heart pumps oxygen to 75 trillion cells from top of body to tips of toes

5 oxygen transfers from blood to muscle via capillaries

Take this quick test

You can get an indirect measure of your cardiorespiratory fitness simply by holding your breath. Sit up straight and take a few deep breaths. Then, using a stopwatch, see how long you can hold your breath. You don't want to strain or get "bug-eyed."

If you cannot hold your breath for at least 60 seconds, it is likely that there is a significant amount of residual carbon dioxide in your body. This affects the acid/alkaline balance of the body, and increased acid levels contribute to illness and disease.

By now, you're probably realizing that exercise is not optional. There is simply no other way to build and maintain muscle; no other way to strengthen your heart and deliver sufficient oxygen to the cells of your body. The Internet is awash with products purporting to alkalize your body, when this can be done for free by exercising.

Accurate but Irrelevant

Today, we are frequently faced with accurate but irrelevant information. When Natalie was in her residency, there was a case discussion regarding a patient with poor respiratory function. The teaching physician handed the chart to Natalie's colleague who recommended a series of tests to evaluate lung capacity, expiratory volume and blood CO_2/O_2 exchange. "That's an accurate diagnostic path," said the mentor, "but what's your treatment plan?" Natalie's colleague replied, "we won't know till we do the tests."

The teaching physician turned to Natalie, who was examining the patient's fingers. "What's your recommendation?" he asked. Natalie replied, "this patient should stop smoking."

In regards to exercise, there is a mountain of accurate but irrelevant information out there. The following is all accurate:

An exercise physiologist will typically divide your program into cardio and resistance exercise, done on separate days. Resistance training should consist of 8 to 12 repetitions (reps) for each major muscle group, at an intensity which is 40% to 80% of a one-rep max (RM). That is one set. After two to three minutes of rest, you are advised to perform two more sets for each muscle group.

For aerobic/cardio training, the standard recommendation is 150 minutes per week of moderate intensity exercise, defined as 46% to 63% of your maximal oxygen uptake (VO2max) for 30 to 60 minutes per session. Further refinements include checking your heart rate. First you find your maximal heart rate (MHR), which is 220 beats per minute minus your age. If you want to lose weight, you are advised to stay in the "fat-burning zone," which is 60% to 70% of your MHR. The "aerobic zone" (70% to 80% of MHR) is for general athletic training and the "anaerobic zone" (80% to 90% of MHR) is for those training for endurance events like a marathon or triathlon.

Accurate, BUT...

This information came in handy when I was helping to train elite athletes. For the other 98% of the population, it is entirely irrelevant, and only serves to confuse, confound and frustrate those who try to do it "by the book." Aren't you relieved?

You know what book you need? The one you're holding. Because much like Natalie's advice regarding the patient with poor lung function, there are simple things that must be done first before launching into a full-scale exercise regime.

1. Improve cellular energy with Metabolic Modifiers

(See Chapter 8.)

2. Get off the couch

66% of North American adults are sedentary; that is, engaged in no consistent exercise program. That shocking fact does not bode well for the suffering and the massive expenditures we face dealing with the consequences of what is now called Metabolic Syndrome.

As we described in Chapter 4, Metabolic Syndrome is insidious. You don't wake up one morning with high blood pressure, diabetes, thick, waxy blood, poor circulation, and an extra 40 pounds of fat on your body. It happens gradually, and it's happening everywhere. The World Health Organization estimates that fully 25% of all the adults on the planet suffer from Metabolic Syndrome, and another 25% are at risk. Every month, Natalie and I are invited to attend conferences on Metabolic Syndrome. Health-care agencies worldwide are asking, "how did this happen?" and the answer is simple: people stopped moving.

We attend conferences where the presenters are overweight and unfit. These scientists and physicians talk about the latest drugs and fail to notice the profound irony of the situation, since drug therapy alone rarely works and improving metabolic fitness always does. When we point this out, we're told that getting people to exercise and change their diet is just too difficult. Natalie and I have dedicated our careers to making it easier. Of course, many people will need drugs to treat their blood pressure, blood sugar, and elevated lipids. But if they don't start moving—in an effective and consistent way—they cannot escape the downward spiral leading to chronic disease, enormous suffering and premature death.

3. Make a plan

Remember that we define "exercise" as being more active today than you were yesterday. But to do that requires that you make time and make a commitment. Many people find that an activity buddy helps; someone to remind you that improving metabolic fitness is a priority.

If getting a human activity buddy is a challenge, we're happy to report that Activity Monitors are a lot more sophisticated than the pedometers we used to hang on our belts. These devices worn on the wrist, ankle, or in a pocket, measure and report your steps, distance, and calories burned. Some even measure sleep duration and quality. Additionally, they automatically synch with your computer or smartphone and create a report to measure your progress and fuel your motivation.

4. Just get started

I know you want to go climb those steps with Rocky, jumping up and down, raising your arms in victory; but remember, slow and steady takes the prize when transitioning out of a sedentary lifestyle.

- Avoid the "Weekend Warrior" Syndrome. Consistent, moderate exercise spread out over the entire week is more beneficial than intense activity concentrated in a day or two. Remember, it's not about "buns of steel" or Terminator biceps.

- Make it moderate. Fatigue and exhaustion can actually slow your progress towards metabolic fitness. Moderate exercise stimulates your metabolism without throwing your body into motivation-killing exhaustion.

- Consistency is more important than intensity. As we've discussed, your genome runs on the principle of efficiency, and predicts your energy needs based upon past experience. If you lead a sedentary life, this cellular "warehouse manager" knows that you don't need much energy, so therefore sends most of the excess calories into storage (to your thighs, for example). So sporadic exercise only confuses the manager. One day he runs out of energy and the next day there's a surplus. The result is that your body experiences no real increase in metabolic efficiency or fat burning.

On the other hand, when you do consistent, moderate exercise, the message to your genome is illustrated in the following Bio-Dialog™.

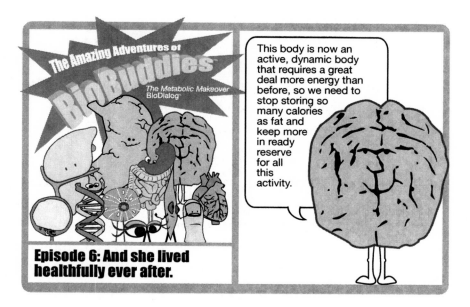

The good news is that this message can be loud and clear even without long, intense exercise sessions. The most important thing is consistency.

Exercising's a walk in the park

Walking is easy, inexpensive (it requires only a good pair of walking shoes), and can be done almost anywhere. Bad weather? Walk in your local shopping mall. Start slow and gradually increase your pace so that you're able to cover two miles in 30 minutes. Then extend the duration to as long as you can. A good 45-minute power walk will do wonders.

Walking is such an efficient exercise because it uses the largest muscles of your body (front and back of your thighs). In fact, you may decide that you like walking so much that you purchase an activity monitor. Some devices signal when you have been sitting for more than 2 hours. And since they register every step you take (even pacing around the office while talking on the phone), the steps add up quickly. Research shows that logging 10,000 steps per day will take you far toward your fitness goals. The 10,000-step target has also been shown to enhance just about any weight-loss program. You'll find yourself checking your monitor midway through the day and adjusting your activity levels — almost automatically — to reach your 10,000-step goal.

NOTE for those over age 40

Metabolic Modifiers can help you regain lost energy and enhance your ability to maintain muscle. But as you go beyond activity into strength training, there's increased risk for injury. A 45-year-old who suddenly finds he can bench-press 180 pounds again may forget that he is pushing that weight with middle-aged joints. And it's not just macho men; women also notice dramatic strength improvements on *The Metabolic Makeover*, and may push too far too fast. It's important, therefore, to go slowly when getting back in shape, and develop an awareness of connective tissue health.

Your skeletal and muscle systems are designed to work together in perfect harmony, allowing your body to maintain just the right mix of flexibility and rigidity. Flexibility enables us to move, dance, run, and jump. Rigidity gives control to these movements so that we don't constantly injure ourselves. Flexibility and rigidity are regulated through the action of joints (which limit the movement of bones) along with ligaments and tendons (which hold joints together and attach muscle to bone).

As we grow older, our joints and connective tissue become dehydrated, much like our skin. Scientists have found a specialized group of compounds known as proteoglycans, which strengthen, hydrate and lubricate tendons, ligaments, and joints. Two well-known proteoglycans are chondroitin and glucosamine.

These can be restored in two ways:

1. Exercise

In true Metabolic Makeover fashion, research shows that exercise stimulates the body to produce new collagen and higher levels of repair and rebuild proteoglycans. This is stunning new data, illustrating one of the pitfalls of research. You see, physiology texts have always asserted that collagen is basically inert. It gets stiff, you get stiff, you die. Turns out, this was true only for the people they were studying, the vast majority of whom were sedentary. In people who remain active, collagen synthesis may take place at any age and the strength of existing collagen can be improved.[4,5]

2. Nutritional support

Chondroitin sulfate has been used as a therapeutic nutrient for centuries. Also available are glucosamine sulfate and N-acetylglucosamine, which perform similar functions.

Other important components of a connective tissue support program include boron, silica, vitamin C, vitamin D, vitamin K, calcium, magnesium and manganese. These substances can sometimes be found in a single tablet or capsule. There is also evidence that collagen synthesis can be increased with nutritional supplements that provide either a high concentration of aloe polysaccharides, or Type-II collagen derived from chicken cartilage.

THE NEXT LEVEL: STRENGTH TRAINING
In order to maximize the benefit of all the exercise you're getting, you need to increase your upper-body strength. Exercises like walking, jogging, tennis, basketball, and racquetball emphasize the major-muscle groups in the legs and provide relatively little benefit to the upper body.

> Sixty-five percent of your muscles are above the waist.

Because these are probably your most underdeveloped muscles, your upper body is the easiest place to build muscle mass quickly. We're not talking about pumping-iron kind of muscles; rather building muscle tone. Research shows that using light weights (five to ten pounds to start) can effectively and efficiently strengthen arm, chest, back, and shoulder muscles. For best results, do your strength training on alternate days to give muscles time to recover.

Get Help

For years, I tried to write out careful instructions for weight training. I reviewed dozens of videos and recommended the best. Still people went out and hurt themselves. I've concluded that it is absolutely essential to use the guidance of an exercise professional, at least for a few sessions. A certified expert will help you set realistic goals and most important, show you safe techniques for each exercise. Whether you're using hand weights, machines, or a combination of both, there is simply no substitute for professional guidance. This technical assistance is often included with health-club membership fees. If you have the financial means, you may want to sign up for personal training, in which case a trainer will stay with you throughout your workout, watching, correcting, and guiding you through each phase of your program.

The Bottom Line

The question everyone asks is, "how much exercise do I need to do in order to stay fit?" Everyone either wants a number to shoot for, or a reason to quit.

So we went looking for a number, and they were not hard to find. Every health agency, fitness trainer, sports medicine website, gym newsletter, and physiology textbook published a number. And they were all different.

We went to medical literature looking for the definitive research. We found scores of studies and they were all different. It's not that these scientists were all doing something wrong; they were just doing different things right. In other words, some measured Total Energy Expenditure (TEE) others measured exercise and non-exercise activity (NEAT) while others measured metabolic equivalents (METs).[6,7,8,9,10,11,12,13,14,15,16,17]

After a week of review with nothing close to a consensus, we decided to use a different approach: observation. After all, between us, Natalie and I have treated and counseled more than twenty thousand individuals. What was the amount and type of exercise that produced the best long-term results?

DRUM ROLL...

WHATEVER YOU FIND THAT YOU CAN DO

CONSISTENTLY

FOREVER.

We want you to think of exercise as a signal to your genome. And that message has to be consistent. If you are mostly sedentary, and exercise on weekends, not only will the benefit be minimal, but the experience will be rather disappointing. That's because your genome, sensing that you are sedentary, dialed down (or turned off) a number of energy-producing pathways. These include the enzymes and transport proteins required to utilize fat as an energy source, as well as the exchange rate of oxygen and carbon dioxide in the lungs.

Then on the weekend, when you want to be active, all of these pathways don't instantly up-regulate to produce an abundance of energy. So you don't really get the feeling of invigoration that you were looking for. It's more like exhaustion, which leads you to think (and this is totally wrong): "I'm too [insert one: old / fat / out of shape] for this." Or even worse, "I'm a bad person."

You're never too old to be active. You may have some musculoskeletal challenges that need to be addressed with regenerative nutrition, but it's not about age; it's about sending a consistent message to your genome, and that message is:

"This is an active body. It requires efficient energy pathways to burn fat and fuel an active lifestyle. What's more, this body requires stronger muscles and improved lung function to meet the needs of regular exercise."

Pop Quiz

Where does this message come from?

A. Your intention

B. Your purchase of exercise equipment

C. Consistent exercise

Tick tock, tick tock...

Buzzer sound...

Answer: C: Consistent exercise.

Thus, the amount of exercise required to maintain physical fitness is:

WHATEVER YOU FIND THAT YOU CAN DO CONSISTENTLY... FOREVER.

For Natalie and me, that turned out to be about five minutes per day.

What? You have got to be kidding.

Come on, what's the number one excuse that people have for not exercising? "I don't have time." Today, everyone is pressed for time. I'm not going to go into the remarkable irony that technology was supposed to give us more free time, but instead created a culture where everything is 24/7, including the work that we're expected to perform. Add to that, the incredible time-sucking technologies like Internet, social media, 500 channel TV and movies on demand... and exercise suddenly disappears from our schedule.

I don't think that's going to change any time soon. In fact, Internet addiction is now a college psychology course...where 95% of the students are addicted to their smartphones. Ha!

Thus, we need to start thinking of ways to get the most benefit in the shortest amount of time. How does 5 to 10 minutes sound to you? You can work up to that. The technique is called by different names, including cross training, maximal training and High Intensity Interval Training (HIIT). These techniques utilize a simple but profound physiologic truth: you can shorten the duration of your workout by increasing the intensity. Why is that?

Cardio-respiratory training is a function of increased oxygen utilization. We keep hearing about heart rate, but that is only a reflection of the muscle's demand for oxygen. With higher intensity exercise, you reach maximal oxygen utilization (also known as VO2Max) very quickly. Compare that to a person walking on a treadmill. Both are considered a cardio workout, but the treadmill walker will use only a fraction of the oxygen compared to someone doing high-intensity intervals. Thus, the person doing the higher intensity exercise will achieve greater benefit in a shorter period of time.

"Intervals" are different exercises that work different muscle groups, and there are literally hundreds of options to choose from. The time-saving advantage derives from the fact that you do these short (20 to 60 second) movements at your maximum intensity, followed by a brief 10 to 60 second rest, before going into the next interval.

The Tabata Technique

High Intensity Interval Training (HIIT) has been around for years, but Dr. Izumi Tabata, a researcher working with elite Japanese athletes, devised a remarkably-effective protocol—pushing his athletes through eight or more 20/10 cycles of high-intensity exercise. His paper, published in 1996, astounded the exercise physiology community, because his group achieved so much in so little time. Since then, Tabata and other HIIT techniques have been shown to be effective for gaining muscle, losing fat and improving cardio-respiratory fitness.

The Tabata 20-second work/10-second rest program can be done with just about any exercise that can be performed in multiple sets. So push-ups, sit-ups, pull-ups, light weights, bands...what stays constant is the protocol—20 seconds of all-out effort followed by 10 seconds of recovery. That's not a lot of rest and that's part of the secret of getting the MOST out of four minutes of exercise. What I like to do is select four exercises that work a variety of muscle groups, and repeat that twice for a total of eight sets.

Fine-tuning

Your four exercises should allow for opposing muscle groups to alternate between resting and working. Push-ups (upper body) could be followed by squats (lower body). Sit-ups could be followed by jumping jacks. This, plus the 10-second rest, allows for the muscles to recover enough to maintain proper form and technique. Tabata should never be sloppy.

You might also like to follow a very active exercise (knee lifts, for example) with a static interval such as stationary plank or ab crunches.

**ARE YOU READY
TO GET THE BEST
4-MINUTE WORKOUT
YOU'VE EVER HAD?**

Example:

A. Push-ups for 20 seconds

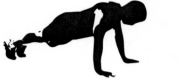

Rest: 10 seconds

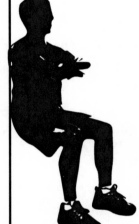

B. Wall sit for 20 seconds
Rest: 10 seconds

C. Jumping jacks for 20 seconds
Rest: 10 seconds

D. Ab crunch for 20 seconds
Rest: 10 seconds

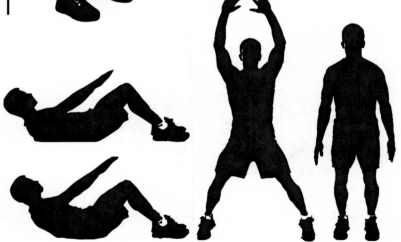

Repeat A,B,C,D for a total of FOUR MINUTES.

There are more than 50 Tabata-style workouts available on YouTube, many that use only the resistance of your own body weight.

No special equipment, no trips to the gym. No excuses.

The secret to the fast results people are seeing is that the Tabata technique is FAR MORE EFFECTIVE than steady-state exercise, whether that's running, walking or biking. Tabata uses what are called type II muscle fibers, which are responsible for definition. High-intensity techniques have other advantages over steady-state. They stimulate testosterone production in men, DHEA and growth hormone in women, and all of that (together with Metabolic Modifiers) helps build exercise tolerance. That means it quickly gets easier and more enjoyable, and that's motivating!

If you WANT to run for an hour, great. If you WANT to work out in a gym, fantastic. But if you're like the VAST majority of adults in North America, you're not going to do that for the rest of your life.

Tabata is the everyday workout, which for me is the all-time best technique. Why? Partly because it's so flexible and partly because I cannot look at the guy in the mirror and tell him that I don't have four minutes.

Importantly, Tabata can be adjusted to ANY fitness level. And don't forget, we ALWAYS recommend consulting with your doctor before starting an exercise program.

I want to introduce an important concept known as hormesis. Simply put, it describes the astounding ability of the human body to adapt to stress. And that includes all kinds of stress: biochemical, physical, and emotional.

In regards to exercise, of course, we're talking about the physical stress that is experienced by the muscles, tendons, ligaments, joints, and bones. As Stephen often points out, we human beings have survived through long periods of tremendous physical stress. So, you would imagine that the human body has evolved some rather intricate and remarkable hormetic responses.

Some are obvious. When you exercise, muscle strength increases. Exercise long enough and the muscles even increase in size to accommodate that stress. Everyone also knows that weight-bearing exercise is important for maintaining strong bones. But we are now learning about hormetic responses to exercise that go far beyond bones and muscles. And along with this new information, comes the realization that some of the things athletes have been doing for decades is entirely wrong.

For example, the free-radical theory of aging that predominated before Stephen's metabolic damage and repair model, led athletes to believe that they should take high doses of antioxidants after exercise. After all, the energy required for strenuous exercise produces huge amounts of free radicals. The idea was that high dose vitamin C and E would mop up those nasty free radicals and speed recovery.

Turns out that was a bad idea. Research published in 2009 demonstrated that taking 1,000 mg of vitamin C and 400 iu of vitamin E actually prevented the normal hormetic response to exercise.[18] Exercise, in other words, is something that evolution strongly favors and produces a comprehensive response that includes a raft of antioxidants produced by a variety of cells in the muscles, liver, and lungs. Oral ingestion of vitamin C and E blunted that response. What's more, these vitamin supplements also abolished the improvement in insulin sensitivity that normally accompanies exercise.

The bottom line: get your antioxidants mainly from a highly-varied natural-foods diet and whole-food concentrates. Subsequent research has shown that whole-food concentrates do in fact assist the body's comprehensive hormetic response to exercise.[19]

Here's another important bit of information. How many of the people in your gym are taking NSAIDS (non-steroidal anti-inflammatory drugs?) There are about 30 of these drugs on the market including: Aspirin (e.g., Anacin®, Excedrin®), Ibuprofen (e.g., Motrin®, Advil®), Naproxen (e.g., Aleve®, Naprosyn®), Sulindac (e.g., Clinoril®), Celecoxib (e.g., Celebrex®), and Indomethacin (e.g., Indocin®). When you take NSAIDS, research shows that it prevents the normal hormetic response in tendons and ligaments.

Think about that. One of the main reasons for exercise is to strengthen connective tissue. When tendons are stressed during exercise, they initiate a repair process that includes increased collagen synthesis. We now know that NSAIDS prevent this from happening.[20] But here's some good news. Exercise stimulates collagen synthesis through a number of signaling molecules, mainly IGF-1.[21] IGF-1 declines with advancing age, but there is a reliable way to increase IGF-1 at any age—and thereby strengthen all connective tissue, including tendons, ligaments, muscles and bones.

TIP #1: Forgo the anti-inflammatory drugs and go with a Metabolic Modifier that increases IGF-1.

What is that marvelous and critically important Metabolic Modifier to increase IGF-1?

A. Creatine

B. Fish oil.

C. DHEA

Answer: C. DHEA.

Tip # 2: There are a number of medicinal plants that naturally reduce inflammation, enabling many people to avoid taking NSAIDS. These include scutellaria Repair, acacia, compounds from hops (botanical name humulus), quercetin, boswellia serata, and curcumin (derived from the turmeric root).

MORE MAXIMAL TRAINING OPTIONS

As we've explained, the primary advantage of Maximal Training is time efficiency, and various companies have developed total-body exercise machines designed to work both the upper and lower body simultaneously. The NordicTrack® Ski Machine is an excellent example, and there are numerous rowing machines that utilize leg and arm resistance at the same time. My favorite is the Rowbike.

I have to say, however, that Natalie and I could not stay as fit as we are without our ROM (short for Range of Motion) Time Machine. This is a two-station row and stair-climb machine that combines all 3 aspects of a complete exercise regimen: cardio-respiratory, resistance, and flexibility. In about 8 minutes, you work more than 50% of your muscles through as much as 80% of their range of motion. Compare that to a treadmill workout that uses about 25% of your muscles through perhaps 20% of their range of motion.

We even find that it's effective to do just a 4-minute upper body workout in the morning before work, and the following morning, perform the 4-minute lower body stair-climb. Tabata, powerwalking hills or the ROM Machine... one way or the other, we rarely let a day go by without at least 4 minutes of Maximal Training.

Our Final Pitch: Do it for your brain

Interestingly, we have found that some people are not terribly motivated by looking good or even feeling energetic. But everyone wants to maintain normal brain function, and fear of dementia is the # 1 concern for the vast majority of people over 60. So, remember when we said that exercise improves everything? Well, new research shows that it can improve cognition and may even help prevent Alzheimer's and Parkinson's disease.[22,23,24]

Natalie note

Prescribing information for doctors states that UP TO 25% of people taking antidepressant drugs gain weight as a result. I would argue that only about 25% of patients do NOT gain weight on these drugs. Clinical data suggests that they stimulate carbohydrate cravings and reduce exercise tolerance. Swell.

To keep the weight gain from affecting drug sales, pharma-oriented websites tell patients that keeping the pounds off is their responsibility since only "healthy eating and exercise help control your weight gain." They conclude with statements like, "If you cannot control your weight with reduced calories and regular exercise, the psychoactive medication to help overcome your depression is far more important."

I'm certainly in favor of treating depression, but in fact, exercise is as effective as drug therapy in improving mild to moderate depression. And the benefits of exercise last longer. I'm not saying that people should stop taking their prescribed drugs. But this is certainly a worthwhile topic to discuss with your doctor before starting drug therapy.

Doctors are information oriented. Print out a few studies to bring to your next visit. In one study, researchers compared the effects of 30 minutes of treadmill walking with 30 minutes per day of quiet rest in a group of men and women recently diagnosed with depression.

The results showed that both groups reported improvements in tension, anger, depression, and fatigue. But only the exercise group reported actually feeling good, as measured by improved scores on "vigor" and "well-being." [25]

We now know that a combination of cardio (aerobic) exercise plus resistance training appears to be the most effective strategy for improving mood.[26,27] Another side effect, of course, is that exercise improves sleep quality, which is known to enhance mood throughout the day.

Summary

1. Looking at how energy is created, stored and used, it is estimated that a fit person produces and experiences about 40 times the energy of an unfit person.

2. The key here is muscle mass, because the quantity and quality of muscle determines, more than any other factor, how much energy is available to you on a daily basis. And there is only one way to increase muscle quality (the number of mitochondria per cell)... regular exercise.

3. Most people lose muscle as they age. This condition, known as sarcopenia, is not inevitable. *The Metabolic Makeover* can prevent and even reverse sarcopenia.

4. Since the #1 excuse that people have for not exercising is "I don't have time," it is important to design a program that produces the greatest benefit in the shortest amount of time. High intensity interval training (HIIT) provides both cardiorespiratory and resistance benefits in 5 to 10 minutes a day.

Endnotes

1 Demontis F, Piccirillo R, Goldberg AL, Perrimon N. The influence of skeletal muscle on systemic aging and lifespan. Aging Cell. 2013 Jun 26. doi: 10.1111/acel.12126.

2 Liao YH, Liao KF, Kao CL, Chen CY, Huang CY, Chang WH, Ivy JL, Bernard JR, Lee SD, Kuo CH. Effect of dehydroepiandrosterone administration on recovery from mix-type exercise training-induced muscle damage. Eur J Appl Physiol. 2012 May 16.

3 Jakubowicz D, Beer N, Rengifo R. Effect of DHEA on cyclic guanosine monophosphate in Men of advancing Age. Annals of the New York Academy of Sciences 1995; 774:312-315.

4 Langberg H, Skovgaard D, Petersen LJ, Bulow J, Kjaer M. Type I collagen synthesis and degradation in peritendinous tissue after exercise determined by microdialysis in humans. J Physiol (Lond) 1999 Nov 15;521 Pt 1:299-306

5 Rennie MJ. Teasing out the truth about collagen. J Physiol (Lond) 1999 Nov 15;521(Pt 1):1

6 Pate RR, Pratt M, Blair SN, Haskell WL, Macera CA, Bouchard C, Buchner D, Ettinger W, Heath GW, King AC. et al. Physical activity and public health. A recommendation from the Centers for Disease Control and Prevention and the American College of Sports Medicine. JAMA. 1995;273:402–407. doi: 10.1001/jama.273.5.402.

7 World Health Organization. Global recommendations on physical activity for health. 2010.

8 Garber CE, Blissmer B, Deschenes MR, et al. Quantity and quality of exercise for developing and maintaining cardiorespiratory, musculoskeletal, and neuromotor fitness in apparently healthy adults: guidance for prescribing exercise. Med Sci Sports Exerc. 2011;43(7):1334Y59.

9 Office of Disease Prevention & Health P; US Department of Health and Human Services. 2008 Physical Activity Guidelines for Americans. 2008.

10 Irwin ML, Yasui Y, Ulrich CM, Bowen D, Rudolph RE, Schwartz RS, Yukawa M, Aiello E, Potter JD, McTiernan A. Effect of exercise on total and intra-abdominal body fat in postmenopausal women: a randomized controlled trial. JAMA. 2003;289:323-330.

11 McTiernan A, Sorensen B, Irwin ML, Morgan A, Yasui Y, Rudolph RE, Surawicz C, Lampe JW, Lampe PD, Ayub K, Potter JD. Exercise effect on weight and body fat in men and women. Obesity (Silver Spring) 2007;15:1496–1512.

12   Elliot DL, Goldberg L, Kuehl KS. Effects of resistance training on excess post-exercise O2 consumption. J Appl Sports Sci Res. 1992;6:77Y81.

13   Slentz CA, Aiken LB, Houmard JA, Bales CW, Johnson JL, Tanner CJ, Duscha BD, Kraus WE. Inactivity, exercise, and visceral fat. STRRIDE: a randomized, controlled study of exercise intensity and amount. J Appl Physiol. 2005;99:1613–1618.

14   Levine JA, Eberhardt NL, Jensen MD. Role of nonexercise activity thermogenesis in resistance to fat gain in humans. Science. 1999;283:212–214.

15   Ohkawara K, Tanaka S, Ishikawa-Takata K, Tabata I. Twenty-four-hour analysis of elevated energy expenditure after physical activity in a metabolic chamber: models of daily total energy expenditure. Am J Clin Nutr. 2008;87:1268–1276.

16   Yamamura C, Tanaka S, Futami J, Oka J, Ishikawa-Takata K, Kashiwazaki H. Activity diary method for predicting energy expenditure as evaluated by a whole-body indirect human calorimeter. J Nutr Sci Vitaminol. 2003;49:262–269.

17   Clark MA, Lucett S, Corn R, et al. Optimum Performance Training for the Health and Fitness Professional. 2nd ed. Calabasas (CA): National Academy of Sports Medicine. 2004. 201

18   Ristow M, Zarse K, Oberbach A, Klöting N, Birringer M, Kiehntopf M, Stumvoll M, Kahn CR, Blüher M. Antioxidants prevent health-promoting effects of physical exercise in humans. Proc Natl Acad Sci U S A. 2009 May 26;106(21):8665-70. doi: 10.1073/pnas.0903485106.

19   Braakhuis AJ, Hopkins WG, Lowe TE. Effects of dietary antioxidants on training and performance in female runners. Eur J Sport Sci. 2013 Apr 20.

20   Christensen B, Dandanell S, Kjaer M, Langberg H. Effect of anti-inflammatory medication on the running-induced rise in patella tendon collagen synthesis in humans. J Appl Physiol. 2011 Jan;110(1):137-41. doi: 10.1152/japplphysiol.00942.2010.

21   Kjaer M, Langberg H, Heinemeier K, Bayer ML, Hansen M, Holm L, Doessing S, Kongsgaard M, Krogsgaard MR, Magnusson SP. From mechanical loading to collagen synthesis, structural changes and function in human tendon. Scand J Med Sci Sports. 2009 Aug;19(4):500-10. doi: 10.1111/j.1600-0838.2009.00986.x.

22   Baker LD, Frank LL. Effects of Aerobic Exercise on Mild Cognitive Impairment. Archives of Neurology, Jan 2010, University of Washington School of Medicine, Seattle

23 Suzuki T, Shimada H, Makizako H, Doi T, Yoshida D, Ito K, Shimokata H, Washimi Y, Endo H, Kato T. A randomized controlled trial of multicomponent exercise in older adults with mild cognitive impairment. PLoS One. 2013 Apr 9;8(4):e61483.

24 Demontis F, Piccirillo R, Goldberg AL, Perrimon N. The influence of skeletal muscle on systemic aging and lifespan. Aging Cell. 2013 Jun 26. doi: 10.1111/acel.12126.

25 Bartholomew, J. Medicine & Science in Sports & Exercise, 2005; vol 37: pp 2032-2037. News release, University of Texas at Austin.

26 Stanton R, Reaburn P, Happell B Is cardiovascular or resistance exercise better to treat patients with depression? A narrative review. Issues Ment Health Nurs. 2013 Jul;34(7):531-8. doi: 10.3109/01612840.2013.774077

27 Loprinzi PD.Objectively measured light and moderate-to-vigorous physical activity is associated with lower depression levels among older US adults. Aging Ment Health. 2013 Jun 3.

Chapter Ten

MEDICAL MAKEOVER

Your physician as your wellness partner
by Natalie Kather, M.D.

Health care in America is changing. I'm not talking about acts of Congress, or insurance overhauls, but rather how patients and doctors relate to each other. For decades, as health care became corporatized and over-regulated, we doctors were pushed into cubbyholes called "specialties." In part, this was due to the astounding amount of information we were expected to learn, along with a constant stream of new drugs and therapies to evaluate.

Office visits became narrow-focused, which made things very efficient for insurance companies. Doctors were told that an office visit was 9 to 11 minutes. If an unrelated issue came up, the patient was simply referred to another specialist. In this fragmented approach, however, underlying metabolic issues were never addressed. Often, they went unnoticed. Without a true integration of information, understanding, and awareness, health care was reduced to merely matching the presenting symptom to the appropriate drug.

I'm happy to say that most doctors really want to have a partnership relationship with their patients. We went to medical school to be healers, not merely drug providers. So when a patient comes in and informs me that they are highly motivated to obtain and maintain optimum health, I celebrate that and welcome them into a healing partnership. This takes work on both sides, and the change I'm seeing in health care is that more and more doctors are looking for motivated patients, and more patients are looking for what is now being called complimentary or integrative medicine.

A motivated patient is one who wants to take responsibility for their health and who understands that, while drugs are often necessary and life-saving, no one has a statin, lisinopril, indomethacin or bisphosphonate deficiency. Considering that the majority of North American adults over 40 are on at least one prescription drug (and the average 65-year-old is on six), it is essential that we learn to work together to make any necessary adjustments as your metabolic health improves.

YOU ARE THE LEADER OF YOUR MEDICAL TEAM.

You now know that optimal health requires physical fitness and that you simply cannot obtain and maintain physical fitness without a highly efficient metabolism. To achieve this, I suggest that you think of creating a Metabolic Makeover team that is in line with your vision and goals. You know your body better than anyone. You are the one that makes all the choices for the care, feeding, exercise and nurturing of your body. Putting together your Metabolic Makeover team will mean choosing providers that understand your fitness goals. You want providers who can do more than say: "you're normal" or "learn to live with it."

My own personal health-care team includes: a nutritionally-oriented medical doctor, chiropractor and massage therapist. I am quite fortunate to live with a nutritional biochemist and human performance expert. When Stephen reminds me that it only takes 4 minutes to do a Tabata workout, I'm grateful that he reminds me to care for myself. As a loving couple, we care for ourselves so we'll live a long, healthy life together.

Some people are better served by a larger health-care team. For a person who suffered a heart attack, ideally the team would include a metabolically-oriented cardiologist, a registered dietician, cardiac rehab specialist and a massage therapist. In building your team, research how providers address your concerns. I can't think of a single malady where diet and exercise don't play a significant role.

A metabolically-oriented physician seeks to address underlying problems. For example, if a person complains of Seasonal Affective Disorder (SAD), fatigue, and low mood that are worse during the winter, symptom-based and metabolically-oriented providers address this differently. A symptom-based approach—which was my medical school and Family Medicine residency training—offers the prescription drug bupropion (eg Welbutrin®) as it has FDA approval for the treatment of Seasonal Affective Disorder.

A symptom-based naturopath may offer St. John's Wort or 5-Hydroxytryptophan as treatment options. A metabolically-oriented physician on the other hand will think differently: "Hmmm, let's see. The person doesn't feel well without consistent sunlight, so let's check vitamin D levels!" And sure enough, the person will have less-than-optimal serum levels of vitamin D. Supplementing the diet with Vitamin D3 to optimal levels not only resolves the person's fatigue and mood decline, but now the muscles, heart, lungs, bone, brain, skin, breasts, colon, immune system, and prostate are all healthier too.

To help find metabolically-oriented providers in your area, talk to friends and co-workers who have health-care providers that help them with issues like nutrition, exercise and hormone balancing. Contact local compounding pharmacies that can direct you to physicians who practice metabolic medicine. Learn about the background of the provider. What is his or her motivation for pursuing additional training to become metabolically oriented?

I was motivated to pursue metabolic medicine because symptom-based medicine had failed me. My hypothyroidism had been missed by at least six physicians. Finally, at a metabolic endocrinology seminar, I learned that one can have "normal" lab values and still suffer with low-functioning thyroid. Correcting that changed my life.

The Intake Form

Once you have your team together, or at least selected a physician, think about how you want the medical visit to go. At my clinic, we have intake forms for the client to complete about their medical history and current state to help me understand their needs and issues. Spend time with this intake form, because it will determine—at least for the first visit—how your doctor relates to you.

The intake form offers a list of questions called the Review of Systems. Usually these are easy to answer by checking off a "yes" or "no" box. The form will also ask you to list all the medications and their dosages, all of your supplements that you take, all the hospitalizations and surgeries you've had. Social history details include smoking, caffeine use, alcohol use and street/recreational drugs use, your career, and perhaps other details about your lifestyle. So you can see that trying to create an effective intake form sitting in the waiting room 10 minutes before your visit is simply impossible.

You might be saying, "That's not fair. Why can't I have a lengthy conversation with my doctor?" Two reasons: first, your doctor doesn't have time for a lengthy conversation and, take it from me, most patients do not have the ability to quickly and accurately describe their medical history, current situation, and goals for the future.

Thus, I urge you to fill out and submit the intake form before you walk into the clinic. Think of this intake form as if it was one of those on-line match-making sites. After all, you are about to enter into a relationship. Include your insights and observations. Did your fatigue begin after a major life stress? Did your strength and stamina decline as you turned 45?

Remember that physicians are written-word oriented. Medical school training tends to select out for those individuals who are good at reading. Many clients provide me with prior laboratory results or chart notes from other providers. Word processing makes it easy to write your observations and concerns, but even hand-written lists for your doctor are useful, such as a record of blood pressures at home or a list of current medications and supplements.

Written descriptions are usually much clearer than a verbal explanation. It is not unusual for me to hear statements like this: "My 63-year-old mother died after having three heart bypasses by the time she was 62, I was only 26 but my brother was 32, so I was worried when my blood pressure was 160 at my third physical therapy visit and I haven't had a menstrual period in 3 months."

This person's stream-of-consciousness statement has very important information in it, but it is difficult and time-consuming for a physician to organize it in a way that best serves the patient. Use the intake form.

Beyond the Written Word

Before your visit, it is also useful to speak with the office manager or Physician Assistant. Ask them if the doctor would be willing to watch a short video prior to the visit that you can shoot with your smartphone or video recorder. These are especially helpful if you are anxious about talking with your physician in person. It should be no longer than 5 minutes.

Please prioritize your concerns and think about how much time is available. Is this visit set for 5 minutes? 20 minutes? 1 hour? The scary concerns should be noted at the very start of the visit... not 4 minutes after it ends.

Communicate

Now that you have given good thought about your health and produced a concise and prioritized intake form, with or without a video, let's talk about how your doctor's brain works to organize data. This is how your physician and your insurance company organize information about your medical concerns.

What symptom(s) do you want to address? Or what is the reason you seek medical care?

That's right. In collecting information about you, even a metabolically-oriented physician asks about symptoms. The difference however, is that the treatment goal is to not only resolve the unwanted symptoms, but to address the underlying cause. Some examples of metabolically-oriented symptoms include:

- High cholesterol
- High blood pressure
- Fatigue, weakness, increased fat, decreased muscle
- Increased waist size
- Slow thinking even after starting a thyroid hormone prescription
- Dizzy and lightheadedness if not eating every 2 hours
- Hair loss, dry skin
- Hot flashes, heat and cold intolerance
- Palpitations, chest pains, chest aches, racing heart, shortness of breath

Regarding these last symptoms, you should give details: When did this start? How long does it last? Does the symptom come and go or is it constant?

At the Doctor Visit

Now, I want to give a few examples of valuable patient communication. Let's choose three common complaints: high cholesterol, high blood pressure and fatigue.

Cholesterol:

"I was first diagnosed with high cholesterol five years ago when I was 30 lb heavier. It improved when I lost weight, but it's been increasing again for the last year—and I've also gained 10 lb in the last year."

"Another doctor prescribed a cholesterol-lowering drug, but I want to learn more about its possible side effects before I start it."

"I took a cholesterol drug five years ago but had to stop it because it made my body ache."

Blood pressure:

"My blood pressure has been high for 10 years. I now take three medications for it because it seems to stay a problem."

"My blood pressure is lower before a meal and very high after I eat, especially if I eat pasta."

"My sister takes blood-pressure medication. My dad had a stroke when he was 65 and he's now 72 years old."

Fatigue:

"For three years now I have no motivation. I have to make myself get things done. It got even worse last year after I had my baby."

"I have started taking acetyl-L-carnitine and alpha lipoic acid. My weight gain has stopped and my energy is better. I have started exercising more."

"I feel better when I don't eat dairy and wheat, but I love how they taste!"

"I started taking magnesium citrate (500mg at bedtime) to help my sleep and I hear it might help my blood pressure. I stopped using '5 Hour Monster Bull' because it has a lot of caffeine."

Prioritize Prioritize Prioritize

Giving me information about your father-in-law's diabetes is not as important as the results of your colon biopsy. Please consider this approach as the client:

> *"Doctor Kather, I have three questions that I wrote down after I submitted my intake forms to your staff. I read an article in your waiting room and*

want to know more. 1) Would you recommend that I take resveratrol and fish oil to improve my blood vessel health since I have high blood pressure and stiff arteries? 2) Can I take the 5 grams of creatine you recommended at the last visit every day? 3) What are branched chain amino acids and how do I benefit from them?"

Now a thorough answer can be given that details energy metabolism and the benefits of supplementing these nutrients. As a client, you can relax and listen without the anxiety of worrying that you won't be able to ask the questions that are truly important to you.

Some people like to take notes, or at least receive references to where they can learn more about topics. Some have so many questions (and for good reason!) that they may not be able to recall the answers. Some bring spouses and friends to help them understand and recall the answers. Some patients like to tape record our visits together.

When clients begin care at my clinic, they receive a folder. This is for them to keep copies of all lab reports and diagnostic imaging reports that they get from us. We readily acknowledge that the client is the leader of the medical team. We want you to track your progress in your labs, tests, and wellbeing.

Be Educated

Congratulations! You are reading this book, so you have already taken an important step in becoming more knowledgeable about your health. Stephen spent three years crafting this book and checking his information sources multiple times. I'm sure you noticed that *The Metabolic Makeover* is thoroughly referenced, with more than 200 footnotes directing the reader to published biomedical literature. I am particularly impressed by the great effort he made addressing numerous food controversies in Chapter 6. I hope that you find this book to be a valuable tool in your quest for optimal health.

We hear that this is "the information age." But it is also the confusion age, since anyone can say anything on the internet, and many people will believe it. The Internet articles that patients bring me range from reliable information to outlandish nonsense, and I try to steer them to sources like www.PubMed.org. This site is free to the public and is created by the National Institute of Health and the National Library of Medicine. With over 32 million citations from worldwide medical literature, it can be a bit overwhelming, so be sure to limit your search to very specific key words.

Be Compliant

One of my clients who had a particularly stellar response to the metabolic medicine approach, tells the story of our initial patient-physician visits. He explains how he was suffering multiple joint pains and decided to try this metabolic approach. I recommended that he start with his diet. He was to stop eating sugar and other refined, processed carbohydrates. As he recounts the story, he laughs about how at the follow-up visit, I seemed confused about his poor clinical response.

He then confessed that he had not been compliant, and had been unwilling to give up nightly ice cream. So we made a deal. If he would be compliant for 60 days, I would continue to serve as his physician. Otherwise, we were both wasting our time. He agreed, and in less than 30 days, experienced dramatic improvements that went far beyond his joints. Sleep quality improved and because of that, so did his energy and mental clarity. I added a plant-based anti-inflammatory, balanced his hormones, and he ended up coming out of retirement to start a new career!

Ask Your Physician/Partner to Monitor Your Progress

The joke in medical school was that the only course in nutrition was held in the cafeteria every day starting at noon. It's no joke, however, that only 30% of medical schools have a single required course in nutrition.[1] Now, that's nutrition in general. The training provided regarding nutritional supplements is zero.

Lesson: do not ask your doctor for permission to take nutritional supplements. Inform them of your decision to use the products. Explain how you selected the product, give them a list of ingredients, and then ask them to monitor whatever they feel is necessary for you to experience best results. If you are a diabetic, they will certainly want you to test your blood sugar. If you are on blood thinners, they'll want to test your clotting time (known as an INR) five to seven days after you start the supplement. In this way, they serve as your partner, and you gain the benefits of safe and effective nutritional products.

Fortunately, nutritional supplements tend to work gradually. I can't think of a single one listed in this book that has a rapid effect that a physician should worry about. They and you will gain from observing the benefits that you experience.

Summary

1. The default doctor/ patient relationship today is similar to a mechanic and a broken car. The patient walks in with a specific complaint, and the doctor goes into "fix-it" mode.

2. If you want something different (like true health care), you will need to create a partner relationship, starting with the intake form.

3. Your doctor's intake form is extremely important because it determines, to a great extent, how your time with the doctor will be spent.

4. Obtain this form from your doctor's office (often from their website) before your first visit. Be thorough, and add any information you want your doctor to have. This may include a short video.

5. In addition to careful attention to your symptoms, meta-bolically-oriented physicians will look for the underlying cause that produced or perpetuates your problem.

Endnotes

1   Kelly M Adams KM, Lindell KC, Kohlmeier M, Zeisel SH. Status of nutrition education in medical schools. Am J Clin Nutr. 2006 April; 83(4): 941S–944S.

Conclusion

For more than 2 million years, our ancestors lived extremely active lives. After all, during that enormous span of time, if you became sedentary, you perished. Since dead people don't pass on their genes, the forces of natural selection produced a genome that strongly favors—actually requires—movement. These are the genes that you and I inherited, that drive and control every cell in your body.

The life you seek is in your muscles still, because you were made to move. And even though you no longer have to; even though you can eke out 70 plus years without lifting anything heavier than your iPad, I know you want more.

The goal, after all, is optimal health; the state of being where you feel so good that nothing can stop you. And at that point, the breakthrough is self-perpetuating because you just want to do the things that support that state of vitality and deep joy.

This is the upward spiral, where life opens to greater and greater possibilities. It's the experience of waking up in the morning, feeling energized and excited; of suddenly noticing in the middle of a busy day that you feel absolutely terrific.

You can achieve this state. It may take some time, but every day will bring its own rewards. *The Metabolic Makeover* is a lifestyle plan that works. Ask yourself this simple question:

Where do I want to be in 5 years? How about 50?

Now, that last number may require a little more thought, because generally, people don't think in terms of half a century. Truth is, however, I can name three technologies in active development, any one of which will have dramatic life-extension benefits.

1. Stem cell therapy
2. Gene therapy
3. Drugs to stimulate the enzyme telomerase in specific cell types to prevent senescence or cell death

The likelihood of at least one of these technologies becoming widely available in the next 25 years is very high. I'm betting on stem cells. None of these, however, will turn back the clock and make a 70-year-old look 35. But they will allow you to keep what you have, in terms of muscle mass, organ and brain function, and general health. That means right now you have a critically important choice. Maximize and maintain your strength, stamina, vitality, and endurance...or risk the chance of a lifetime, either by becoming too frail or already dead.

Using Your Brain to Build your Body

Your muscles have another enemy other than inactivity. It's called stress. Unmanaged stress—the kind that keeps you up at night or causes anxiety—can weaken or destroy your muscles.

Why would the body do that?

As we learned in Chapter 1, your genome is constantly monitoring your physical and emotional state, in order to ensure your survival. For millions of years that meant not getting killed, which required the genome to develop the fight-or-flight response.

This response has two phases. In what is called episodic stress (face to face with a saber-tooth tiger) the hormone norepinephrine dilates the pupils to improve vision, accelerates the heart rate, and tells the liver to dump fuel (glycogen and fat) into the bloodstream in order to escape the danger.

The second phase kicks in if the stress becomes chronic or long-lasting. This is activated by the hormone cortisol, which sets off panic activity in the brain, heart, blood vessels, liver, gut, and nervous system. It tells the body to start breaking down muscle.

Why? Because in a chronic emergency state, amino acids become a last-ditch fuel.

Today, most people experience episodic and chronic stress on a regular basis. What's more, excess caffeine raises cortisol and interferes with sleep, setting up a vicious cycle where the individual wakes feeling exhausted instead of rested. And what do most people reach for? More caffeine!

TIME OUT!

When was the last time you did nothing at all for an hour? I find it remarkable that most people have a hard time remembering a recent hour when they were not active either with work, recreation or entertainment.

Most of us are "connected" 24/7 with cell phones, pagers, tablets, TVs, and laptops, and assume that's a good thing, because after all, we wouldn't want to miss anything, right?

There's a downside to all this, and you know it. Constant communication adds stress to our lives, and quickly becomes addicting. I have seen people frantically searching for their cell phone as if it was a lost child or beloved pet.

Perspective

For eons, we rested in the sounds of nature—a running stream, chirping crickets, singing birds—what are called primordial sounds. They are literally encoded in our genes, so it's no surprise that listening to these sounds today will lower your heart rate and blood pressure and put you at ease. By contrast, listening to police sirens, traffic noise, and television violence produces anxiety and contributes to illness and disease.

When was the last time you walked through a dense forest? Natalie and I try to experience this on a daily basis, walking a trail from our home to Puget Sound. We do this in an effort to balance our extremely busy lives.

The Pace of Change

For millions of years, the most significant and noticeable change was the passage of time, marked by the seasons. Today, the pace of change in all areas of life is blinding, and it affects us all on some level.

For Natalie and me, it means dealing with new information, which is produced at an astounding rate. Picture the aggregate sum of all scientific information produced from Isaac Newton (1642 – 1727) to the present day. Printed out, it would fill more than four baseball stadiums from home plate to the top of the bleachers. That astronomical amount of information now doubles every 2 ½ years.

Natalie and I deal with that by creating a team of colleagues, each one responsible for a particular specialty. But we still find our schedules increasingly crowded. Everyone we know is dealing with some aspect of rapid and unrelenting change. And of course, that's just the beginning. The Internet, social media and 500-channel TV are all calling for our attention, and we all have one or more jobs to perform.

Just getting to work can be stressful. I used to have a four-minute commute along a tree-lined country road. Then because of the need to expand our research facility, the lab was moved to downtown Seattle. Since Natalie can't move her Olympia clinic, and I have 5 kids in school, I was suddenly faced with a 1 ½-hour commute. That's three hours of my day in heavy traffic. Faced with events like this, it's tempting to cut out things like exercise and periods of stillness, but those are exactly the activities that you cannot do without.

The Value of a Reasoned Retreat

When I speak of retreat, I'm not talking about weekend retreats to the woods, although I'm all in favor of those, too. Such retreats help put things in perspective and give us opportunities to know ourselves and our loved ones better. Nor am I talking about sticking your head in the sand to artificially blind yourself to life's stresses. Blindness does not equal serenity.

What I'm talking about is using our hearts and minds to evaluate whether there are things in our lives that are not serving us, things that are hindering our advancement instead of helping us get where we really want to go. It can be helpful to scan our relationships, work, and habits to evaluate whether they are helping or hurting us. Do they bring a sense of joy and peace to our lives?

You might say that what I'm suggesting is the equivalent of burying your head in the sand, but I don't think it is. My question to you is this: how does it improve your life to know that a ferry boat capsized in a far-off land today killing 356 people? Do you really need to know what a Facebook friend had for lunch? What will you do differently today because of that knowledge? How are you made stronger or how are you now able to contribute to the world, because of the footage you saw on the evening news? You are informed, yes, but so what?

Random bits of information by themselves, robbed of a context in which you are actually able to do something about them, are useless. In reality, the endless barrage of conflict and tragedy from every corner of the earth wears us down, adds to our stress, and creates a feeling of helplessness. I believe we tend to do less in our communities —where it matters—because we're so wrapped up in things that don't matter.

Mindfulness: The Makeover For Your Mind

I'm always surprised when I check into a hotel and find three televisions; one in the room itself, another in the bedroom, and a third... in the bathroom! And it's not only the sheer volume of information that can be sent screaming into my consciousness by these devices. It's the nature, content, and intention of the information.

What if you unplugged yourself from the pop culture idea that you have to know everything that is happening in the world all the time. Take a look at how television and the Internet have commandeered your time and attention and ask yourself if this is helping you become a happier or better person.

The Nature of time

Have you noticed how time changed as you became an adult? In childhood, there was an immediacy of experience that included a remarkable openness to new ideas. As an adult, the way you think about these critical facets of life is colored by years of anxiety about the future and remorse or reverie concerning the past. The result is that many people can hardly focus at all on the most important thing: the present.

Watch yourself as you go through the day and see how much of your attention is firmly fixed on the past or the future. I suggest that this reduces quality of life in subtle but significant ways, because it's only in the present that you can be truly alive. To demonstrate this, I recommend a simple exercise. Remember what a day was like when you were a child, how it stretched across what seems now to be an eternity of activity, play, adventure, meals, and then (forestalled as much as possible) bedtime. A day then was the same 24 hours, and yet today those 24 hours seem to fly by in a flash. I believe the difference is mindfulness.

As children, we were intensely present for almost every activity and event in which we were involved. Part of this intensity was the utter newness of experience, part was the lack of anxiety about the future. And then there was the fact that our lives (at least until we entered school) were not regimented into a clock-oriented schedule. We enjoyed a very primitive relationship with time.

Mindfulness is the practice of being present. We can regain the intense joy and exuberance of youth because it's always there. Mindfulness requires some getting used to. It involves becoming acutely present to every experience. When eating, this means being aware of every mouthful, the subtle nuances of taste and aroma. When showering, this means feeling the caress of hot water, the richness of soap, the nap of the towel. You are wholly engaged in life, with what you have and where you are, as opposed to running on auto-pilot towards some imagined happiness and fulfillment in the future.

With mindfulness, even unpleasant experiences are felt fully and completely. In this way they are robbed of the power they often hold in our consciousness. After all, much of the pain of unpleasant experience is tied to the incredible amount of energy and attention we spend in pre-event anxiety and post-event regret. Being mindful involves understanding that we cannot "unhappen" things that happen. "Go with the flow" is good advice, but makes sense only when you have seen and deeply felt this flow in your life. The practice of mindfulness can reveal the flow in a powerful and life-altering way, enabling you to experience a "slowing down" of time, a shift in your relationship to the people, events, and priorities in your life.

Modern attempts at time management (planners, alarm watches, overnight and same-day mail delivery, faxes, cell phones, endless e-mail, social media, 24/7 goods and services) cannot give us the freedom and sense of ease we yearn for if we are not mindful.

Genuine life experience, in other words, is not just a vibrantly healthy body, but a vibrantly healthy life, which includes peace of mind. Creating (or at least contemplating) a shift in our relationship to time is an important step.

Meditation: It's Not What You Think

People often imagine that meditation is an escape from worldly cares and concerns, a kind of cosmic cocoon. But that's the stereotype. Meditation is a very proactive practice. It will not bury or hide anything. On the contrary, it brings everything up for review. This review, however, is entirely different than your normal obsessing and fear. It is objective and calm, and there is a piercing clarity to the process that quickly brings priorities into focus.

Meditation does more than help you sort things out. The mind, more than anything, desires peace. Meditation provides that experience and helps synchronize your actions with this core desire. The mind responds by creating the insights and awareness you need to remove stress from your life. "Hey, trading commodities is giving me an ulcer. I think I'd rather be a landscape engineer."

Meditation may also help your heart by decreasing risk for cardiovascular disease. A recent study compared a group of subjects with high blood pressure who completed a meditation program with another hypertensive group that took part in a health education course. The people who meditated for 20 minutes twice a day over the 7-month study period experienced a significant reduction in the thickening of their artery walls, indicating a reduction of risk for stroke and heart attack. Those in the health-education group experienced an increase in artery wall plaque buildup. The researchers propose that meditation triggered repair mechanisms that helped clear fatty deposits from the blood vessels.[1]

One Step at a Time

What if you decided to spend 30 minutes to an hour a day doing nothing, literally unplugged? There are any number of tools that can help you make the most of this time. The easiest is to simply sit quietly and observe your breath. This is the simplest meditation technique, used by billions of people for thousands of years. It's effective because it leads the mind to stillness. Biochemically, it reduces stress hormones like cortisol, which fosters repair and rebuild activity throughout the body and brain.

Peace is our natural state. It is only because we force our mind into constant attention to the outside world that we miss out on this critically important experience. Breathing is automatic. You don't try to breathe. And observing your breath has a powerful way of centering the mind.

In this technique, you don't force the breath in any way. You simply observe the breath rising in your belly, rib cage, and upper chest. Watch the exhalation empty first from the upper chest, then rib cage and finally the belly.

After a few minutes, there will be a shift of attention from the breath to what is called awareness. Where this leads does not matter. At first, it might be your task list or some other busy thought. No matter. This is not the time to judge the quality of your thoughts, but to simply watch them come and go. With practice, the mind will become still and true insight will arise. Remember, peace is your true nature. You are simply providing the conditions for this to unfold.

Shared Values

In primitive societies, the individual is an integral and valued member of society, playing a cooperative role in virtually every activity, from building shelter to finding and preparing food. On the other hand, our present society (barely a few centuries old), is oriented around competition for goods and material assets. The illusion is that we are self-sufficient, but in fact we are not. Few of us could survive if we had to gather our own food. Some believe as I do that much of modern angst is our alienation from nature and the increasing dependency on others for survival.

Then there is the ceaseless media drumbeat telling you that your body is not thin enough, your lips not fat enough, your car not fast enough, and your whites not white enough. To the degree that we buy into this, we will run out and buy clothes, automobiles, fragrances, and other consumer goods; chasing the promise that owning such things will make us complete and whole. We become blind to what really matters, but as the saying goes, the best things in life are not things.

So what do we do? We can't go back to a tribal society, but we can become more cooperative. Social media has certainly made us more connected, but I am not sure how much of that is true community. Instead of these virtual communities that result from typing on a keyboard, why not spend more time visiting with your actual neighbors?

We all need tools to manage change, and the best tool is the care and concern of friends. Support from friends, family, and community has been shown to reduce feelings of isolation and produce significant increases in wellness biomarkers. Individuals who enjoy a deep sense of community, either religious, ethnic, or merely geographic, have decreased risk for heart disease and cancer. Community builds immunity.

What does all this mean to you? Perhaps it suggests the need for a shift in your relationship to time from the frantic, time-is-running-out consciousness that prevails in today's society, to a more relaxed experience of life. Remember taking the SAT exam? The pressure was tremendous, not only because the results would determine our college choices, but because there was a time limit. We were trying to beat the clock. Well, put yourself back in that pressure-cooker experience and imagine the test monitor making an announcement ten minutes before the buzzer: "Attention, students: if you need more time, feel free to take another hour to give it your best effort."

That's what mindfulness is all about; giving you more time so that you can get the most from – and contribute the most to – life. Of course, there are still only 24 hours, but mindfulness makes those hours richer and more meaningful.

And finally, I want to acknowledge that making changes in your life is never an easy task. The key, however, is not to get caught up in the distance you have to go. Whether it's losing fat and gaining muscle or learning a meditation technique, progress is made in small, intentional steps. I believe that Natalie and I have provided an accurate map because we've watched and celebrated the success of thousands already. You have more power than you might think. By focusing on the small steps that you can take every day, the progress you make will motivate you to continue your journey and eventually, you can get to wherever you want to go.

THE IMPORTANT THING IS TO SIMPLY BEGIN!

Endnotes

1   Castillo-Richmond A, Schneider R. H, Alexander C. N, Cook R, Myers H, Nidich S, Haney C, Rainforth M, Salerno J. Effects of stress reduction on carotid atherosclerosis in hypertensive African Americans. Stroke 2000 Mar;31(3):568-573.

Index

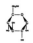

272

CPSIA information can be obtained at www.ICGtesting.com
Printed in the USA
LVOW06s1537120614

389806LV00009B/1349/P